trotman

LAUREL ALEXANDER

Nursing & Midwifery UNCOVERED

Nursing and Midwifery Uncovered
This first edition published in 2004 by Trotman and Company Ltd
2 The Green, Richmond, Surrey TW9 1PL

Editorial and Publishing Team

Author Laurel Alexander
Editorial Mina Patria, Editorial Director; Rachel Lockhart, Commissioning Editor; Anya Wilson, Editor; Bianca Knights, Assistant Editor
Production Ken Ruskin, Head of Pre-press and Production
Sales and Marketing Tom Lee, Commercial Director; Deborah Jones, Head of Sales and Marketing
Managing Director Toby Trotman

Designed by XAB

British Library Cataloguing in Publication Data
A catalogue record for this book is available from the British Library

ISBN 0 85660 963 3

Typeset by Palimpsest Book Production Limited, Polmont, Stirlingshire

Printed and bound in Great Britain by Cromwell Press, Trowbridge, Wiltshire

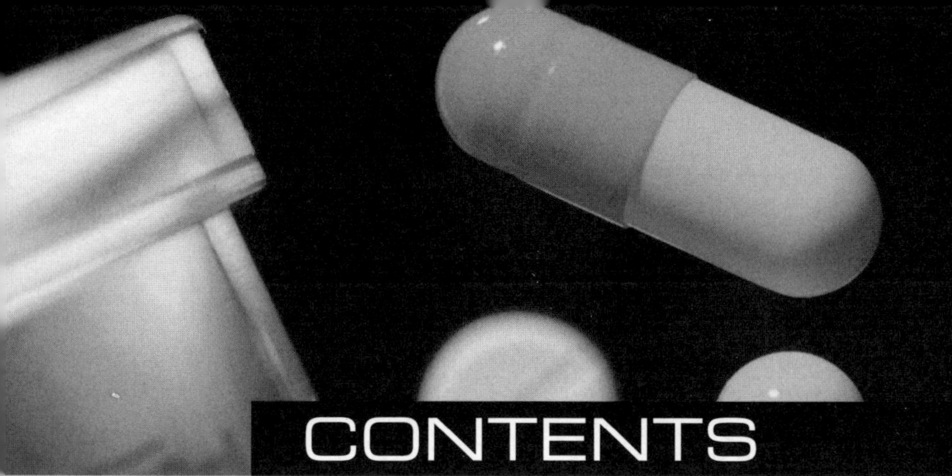

CONTENTS

About the Author

Laurel Alexander works as a complementary breast cancer care therapist with the Royal Sussex County Hospital and has a thriving private practice as a healthcare professional in Brighton. She also teaches courses in counselling skills, assertiveness training, women and health as well as being the Director of Studies for the Diploma in Holistic Stress Management, a course accredited by the National Council of Psychotherapists. She has appeared on TV and radio giving advice on healthcare matters.

Her other books for Trotman include: *Getting into Complementary Therapies*, *Getting into Healthcare Professions*, *Getting into Physiotherapy* and *Medicine Uncovered*. Laurel is also a journalist, with health-related features published in national magazines and professional journals including *Yoga and Health*, *Positive Health*, *Reflexions* (journal of the Association of Reflexologists) and *CancerBACUP*.

Acknowledgements

I would like to thank the Armed Forces, Royal College of Nursing and NHS Careers for their invaluable help.

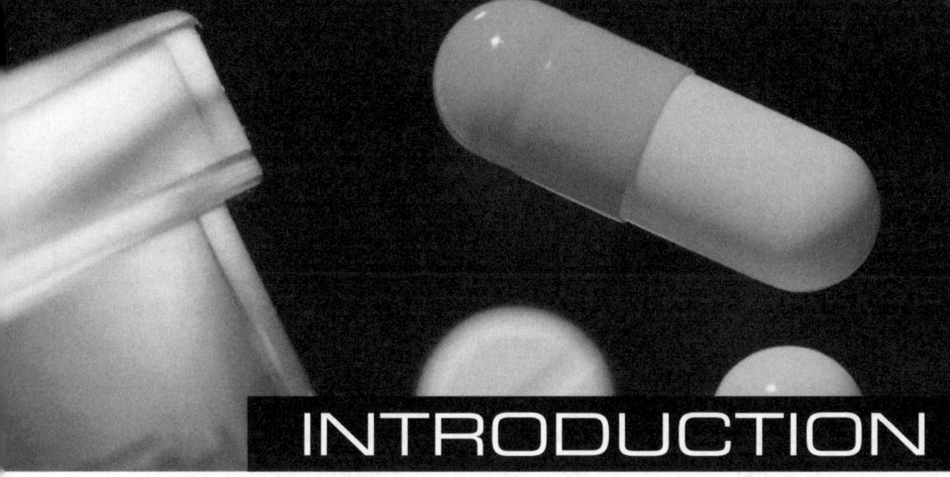

INTRODUCTION

WHAT'S THIS BOOK ABOUT?

To put it simply, this book tells you about careers in nursing and midwifery, where you could work, what you might earn and how you can become a nurse or midwife.

WHAT'S IN IT FOR YOU?

You might be looking for your first career or you might want a change of career. Nursing and midwifery are two of the most fascinating options you could choose to explore. If you like working with people, want to make a difference to their lives in times of anxiety, fancy being paid well and want a job where you know the difference between your Deaver's windows (the spaces in the flesh that hold the guts in position, named after their discoverer, American scientist John Blair Deaver) and your umbilicus (the hole where the feeding tube of the unborn baby joins the body – belly button!) then you must read the rest of this book.

MIDWIFERY

The midwife has been part of the human experience for as long as we know. The ancient Jews called her the wise woman, just as she is known in France as the *sage-femme*, and in Germany, the *weise Frau* and also *Hebamme* or mother's advisor, helper, or friend.

FASCINATING FACT

The term 'midwife' is derived from Middle English 'midwife', or 'with-woman' (J.H. Aveling). The Latin term *cum-mater* and the Spanish and Portuguese term *comadre* have the same meaning: with-woman.

A midwife figures in the Book of Genesis, 35:17: 'And when she [Rachel] was in her hard labour, the midwife said to her, "Fear not, for now you will have another son."' And we find in the Book of Exodus, 1:20 that 'God dealt well with the midwives: and the people multiplied, and waxed very mighty.'

In ancient times and in primitive societies, the work of the midwife had both a technical or manual aspect and a magical or mystical aspect. Hence, the midwife was sometimes revered, sometimes feared, sometimes acknowledged as a leader of the society, sometimes tortured and killed. The midwife had knowledge and skill in an area of life that was a mystery to most people. Since women had no access to formal education, it was widely assumed that the midwife's power must come from supernatural sources, such as an alliance with the devil. During the Middle Ages, up to several million women fell victim to a witch-burning frenzy, many being midwives and healers.

Today, in much of the world, professional midwives are responsible for attending women in labour and birth. In fact, in the countries with the best pregnancy outcomes, midwives are the primary providers of care to pregnant women.

You could become a midwife in the NHS, based in a hospital or the community. Or you might want to be an independent midwife, working in all kinds of environments with women who want a wider range of pregnancy and labour options.

If you would like to be a midwife, you could find yourself working:

- **in an NHS hospital**
- **in a private clinic**
- **in people's homes**

NURSING

Once you have the basic nursing qualifications, you can go anywhere in the world. You could work in the public (NHS) or private sector and you could specialise in a huge variety of conditions.

NURSES OF TOMORROW?

Journalists visited five schools from across the UK to talk to groups of students aged 11–12 and 14–15 about their perceptions of nurses and nursing. Asked what came into their heads when they heard the word 'nurse', one student said 'hospitals', another added 'Red Cross'. A student from Brighton thought of 'surgeries and X-rays'. Another said 'white outfits'. Broader concepts were also offered such as 'injections' and 'medicines'. One young student said it made him think of 'life and death'. Many students referred to 'caring', 'making people comfortable' and 'hardworking'.

Two pupils had particularly insightful views; 'I think nurses reach out to people,' said one, and another commented, 'They make them think something different, they tell them they are not going to die.' Another student said, 'Kind and horrible people. Some nurses can be really kind and they will try to help you, but some others can try to rush you about and be horrible to you all the time.'

What did the students think nurses do? One thoughtful response from an 11-year-old was 'They help the ill and injured and if a patient tells them something in confidence, they do not tell anyone else.' Another student commented, 'I think nurses are more sympathetic than doctors. They give you more attention than doctors.'

When asked the difference between doctors and nurses, a student said 'A nurse would heal people's cuts whereas a doctor would heal them from illness.'

When students were asked to identify famous nurses, the results ranged from Mother Theresa, *Casualty*'s Charlie Fairhead and *Coronation Street*'s Martin Platt together with *Scrubs*, *ER* and 'that gay man from *Casualty*'.

Nursing Standard

Nursing these days is about promoting health as well as treating the sick. A lot of the work community nurses do is about giving local people help, advice and support to improve their own health.

NURSING – A COUPLE OF KEY PLAYERS

Florence Nightingale

The second daughter of William Edward Nightingale and Frances, Florence was named after her birthplace. She grew up in Derbyshire, Hampshire and London, where her family maintained comfortable homes. She was educated largely by her father, who taught her Greek, Latin, French, German, Italian, history, philosophy and mathematics. Throughout her life she read widely in many languages. On 7 February 1837, she believed that she had heard the voice of God informing her that she had a mission, but it was not until nine years later that she realised what that mission was.

Meanwhile, she strove to escape to a life of her own. Her proposal to study nursing was refused, but she was persuaded by the then Lord Ashley to study parliamentary reports and public records relating to health matters and health reformers (such as Edwin Chadwick) and in three years she was regarded by influential friends as an expert on public health and hospitals. Nightingale went on to develop schools of nursing and played a pivotal role in the care of the sick and wounded in the Crimean War, at Scutari. To hear a recording of her voice, click on **www.internurse.com/history/nightingale/nightingale.htm** (internurse.com).

St Camillus of Lellis (1550–1614) (The patron saint of nursing is a man!)

Having been reduced to poverty by heavy gambling, Lellis was employed by the Capuchins of Manfredonia. In 1570 he began to live a life of penance and became a nurse at the hospital of St Giacomo in Rome; he was ordained a priest in 1584. He established a following whose members took a vow to devote themselves to the material and spiritual care of the sick and those suffering from the plague. Camillus of Lellis founded the Ministers of the Sick, and there is a hospital in Northumberland staffed by the Brothers of St Camillus.

When I was about to leave school, a five-minute careers guidance interview clarified what I wanted to 'be' when I left – a nurse. I enrolled in cadet school at a local hospital where I would go to prepare for my career. Way back then (I'm the ripe old age of 45 now), I had visions, encouraged by my mother, of swanning down the road in my red-lined nurse's cape, dispensing grapes down parched throats and wiping fevered brows with cool flannels. But with the contrariness of youth (and when I was skipping school one day), I decided I wanted to be a window dresser in a fashionable clothes shop instead. So down the drain went my mother's fond hopes and any vague dreams I may have had of healing the sick. Only about 20 years later did I step back into those early aspirations and become a healthcare professional. I'm not a nurse but a complementary therapist. I'm not a nurse but I work closely with Macmillan nurses in working with cancer patients. I'm not a nurse but many of my clients are nurses themselves.

I tell you this because if you aspire to be a nurse, there are so many opportunities where you can build on basic nursing qualifications to work in so many different environments, making a real difference in people's lives. Don't just think of nurses on a ward – you're only as limited in your work opportunities as you are in your imagination!

If you would like to be a nurse, you could find yourself working:

- in a hospital ward
- in a university
- in a residential home
- in a hotel
- in a prison
- in a day hospital
- in a community services centre
- in a woman's health centre
- with abortion services
- in a specialist fertility clinic
- with industry/commerce
- with a pharmaceutical company
- in a nursing home
- in people's homes
- on a cruise ship
- on a health farm
- in a children's home
- in a day centre
- in a care home
- with cosmetic surgery patients
- in a GP practice
- in A&E
- on a helpline
- in health centres

- in a clinic
- in a blood donor centre
- with adolescent services
- in outpatients
- in a (boarding) school
- with the Army, Navy or Air Force
- in an outreach capacity
- with air ambulance services
- in oncology
- in an operating theatre
- in a specialist baby unit
- in intensive care
- in a maternity unit
- in a hospice
- in a community rehabilitation unit
- in a secure unit
- in a sexual health clinic

DO YOU HAVE WHAT IT TAKES?

The more questions you can answer yes to, the more likely you are to succeed in a nursing or midwifery career:

- Are you a good self-manager?
- Can you be accountable for your actions?
- Do you enjoy working with people?
- Are you non-judgmental?
- Can you empathise with others?
- Have you the flexibility to juggle the needs of a number of individuals at the same time?
- Can you set people at their ease in pressurised and sometimes difficult circumstances?
- Can you be reassuring to others?
- Could you be confident at handling the distress of carers and family?

- Do you have patience?
- Have you well-developed, flexible communication skills?
- Can you cope with stressful and demanding people?
- Can you show warmth to others?
- Have you good listening skills?
- Can you provide advice and support?
- Have you understanding and intuition?
- Can you be tolerant and objective?
- Are you flexible?
- Are you reliable?
- Have you a mature and responsible attitude?
- Do you have the ability to work independently and as part of a team?
- Are you enthusiastic?
- Do you have mental and physical energy?

Still interested? Fancy your chances as a nurse or midwife? Read on to discover what it's like to work in the public and private sectors.

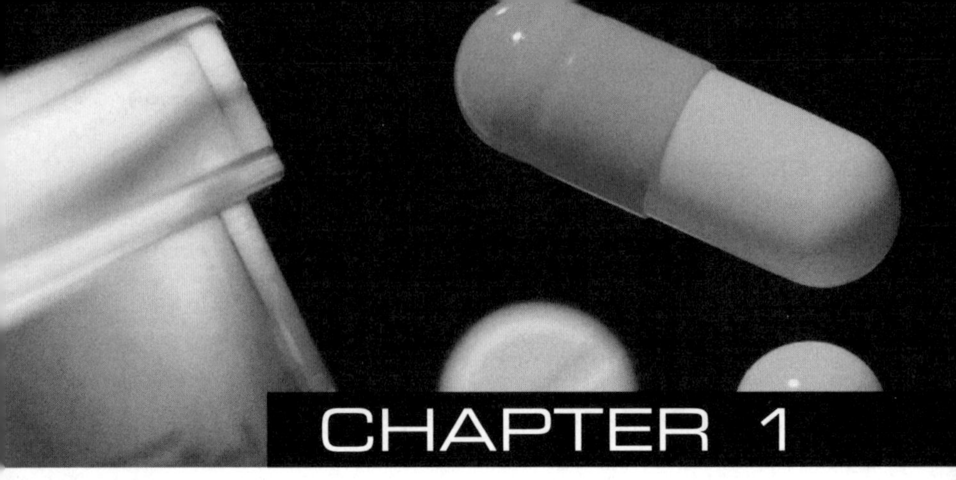

Working in the Public and Private Sectors

Qualify as a nurse or midwife and you can choose to work in the public (NHS) or private sector. Here's what they're both about – and how much you can get paid in each sector.

WORKING FOR THE NHS

The NHS was set up over 50 years ago and is now the largest organisation in Europe.

THE PRE-1948 SCENE AND HEALTHCARE

The same services were available just before the creation of the NHS as afterwards; no new hospitals were built nor were hundreds of new doctors employed. What was different before was that poor people had often gone without medical treatment, relying instead on home remedies or on the charity of doctors who gave their services free to their poorest patients.

Hospital fees: Access to a doctor was free to workers who were on lower pay, but this didn't necessarily include their wives or children, nor did it extend to other workers or those with a better standard of living. Hospitals charged for services, though poorer people would sometimes be reimbursed. The need for free healthcare was widely recognised, but it was impossible to achieve without the support or resources of the state.

Philanthropists and social reformers: Throughout the 19th century, philanthropists and social reformers had tried to provide free medical care for the poor. William Marsden, a young surgeon, opened a dispensary for advice and medicines in 1828. The London General Institution for the Gratuitous Cure of Malignant Diseases – a simple four-storey house in one of the poorest parts of the city – was conceived as a hospital to which the only passport should be poverty and disease and where treatment was provided free of charge to any destitute or sick person who asked for it.

Royal Free Hospital: By 1844 Marsden's dispensary, now called the Royal Free Hospital, was treating 30,000 patients a year. With consultant medical staff giving their services free of charge, and money from legacies, donations, subscriptions and fundraising events, the Royal Free – now rehoused in larger premises – strove to fulfil Marsden's vision until 1920 when, on the brink of bankruptcy, it was forced to ask patients to pay whatever they could towards their treatment.

Municipal hospitals: As well as the charitable and voluntary hospitals, which tended to be mainly for serious illnesses, local authorities in large towns provided municipal hospitals – maternity hospitals, hospitals for infectious diseases like smallpox and tuberculosis, as well as hospitals for the elderly, 'mentally ill' and 'mentally handicapped'.

Mental institutions: People deemed mentally ill or mentally handicapped were locked away in large forbidding institutions, often not for their own benefit but to save other people from embarrassment. Conditions were often so bad that many patients became worse, not better.

Older people: Older people who were no longer able to look after themselves also fared badly. Many ended up in the workhouse – a Victorian institution where paupers did unpaid work in return for food and shelter. Workhouses changed their names to Public Assistance Institutions in 1929, but a stigma remained attached to them.

DEPARTMENT OF HEALTH

The Department of Health is the government department that looks after the health and well-being of the population and is responsible for:

- setting overall direction and leading transformation of the NHS and social care
- setting national standards to improve quality of services
- securing resources and making investment decisions to ensure that the NHS and social care are able to deliver services
- working with key partners to ensure quality of services.

COMMISSION FOR HEALTH IMPROVEMENT (CHI)
The CHI acts as an independent inspectorate to ensure standards set by the Government, through its health policies and National Service Framework, and clinical guidance provided by the National Institute for Clinical Excellence, are met. Local healthcare organisations in the NHS will be reviewed every three or four years. The CHI also has the power to carry out or assist in investigations and enquiries into serious service failures. It helps NHS organisations draw up action plans to tackle problems or areas of weakness, providing expert support and advice drawn from the best service providers. The CHI was set up in October 1999.

STRATEGIC HEALTH AUTHORITIES

In April 2002, 28 new, larger Strategic Health Authorities (SHAs) were set up to develop strategies for the NHS, and to make sure their local NHS organisations were performing well. The new health authorities have a strategic role. They are responsible for:

- developing plans for improving health services in their local area
- making sure national priorities – for example, programmes for improving cancer services – are integrated into local health service plans
- making sure local health services are of a high quality and are performing well
- increasing the capacity of local health services – so they can provide more services.

SHIFTING THE BALANCE OF POWER

Shifting the Balance of Power is the name for the programme of changes that are reforming the way the NHS works. The aim is to design a service centred on patients, which puts them first. It will be faster, more convenient and offer them more choice. The main feature of the change has been to give locally based Primary Care Trusts (PCTs) the role of running the NHS and improving health in their areas. This has also meant creating new Strategic Health Authorities, which cover larger areas and have a more strategic role.

PRIMARY CARE TRUSTS

Primary Care Trusts (PCTs) are at the centre of the NHS and work with local authorities and other agencies that provide health and social care locally to make sure the community's needs are being met. As local organisations, they are best placed to appreciate the needs of their community. For example, PCTs:

- must make sure there are enough services for people in their area and that they are accessible to patients

- must make sure that all other health services are provided, including hospitals, dentists, mental health services, NHS Walk-In Centres, NHS Direct, patient transport (including A&E), population screening, pharmacies and opticians
- are responsible for ensuring health and social care systems work together to the benefit of patients.

PRIMARY CARE
This is the care provided by people you normally see when you first have a health problem. It might be a visit to a doctor or dentist, an optician for an eye test, or just a trip to a pharmacist to buy cough mixture. NHS Walk-in Centres and the phone line NHS Direct are also part of primary care. All the people offering primary care are now managed by the new local health organisations, PCTs.

NHS TRUSTS AND HOSPITALS

NHS Trusts manage hospitals, making sure that they provide high-quality healthcare and that they spend their money efficiently. They also decide on a strategy for how a hospital will develop so that services improve. Trusts employ most of the NHS workforce, including nurses, doctors, dentists, pharmacists, midwives and health visitors as well as others whose jobs are related to medicine – physiotherapists, radiographers, podiatrists, speech and language therapists, counsellors, occupational therapists and psychologists. There are many other non-medical staff including receptionists, porters, cleaners, IT specialists, managers, engineers, caterers and domestic and security staff. Some trusts are regional or national centres for more specialised care. Others are attached to universities and help to train health professionals. Trusts can also provide services in the community, for example through health centres, clinics or in people's homes. Except in emergency cases, hospital treatment is arranged through a GP. This is called a referral.

AMBULANCE TRUSTS

There are 33 ambulance services covering England, which provide emergency access to healthcare. If you call for an emergency ambulance the calls are prioritised into three categories:

- Category A emergencies – which are immediately life-threatening
- Category B or C emergencies – which are not life-threatening.

The control room decide what kind of response is needed and whether an ambulance is required. For all three types of emergency, they may send a rapid response vehicle, crewed by a paramedic, equipped to provide treatment at the scene of an accident. Over the last five years the number of ambulance 999 calls has gone up by a third.

The NHS is also responsible for providing transport to get patients to hospital for treatment. In many areas it is the Ambulance Trust which provides this service.

THE MODERNISATION AGENCY

The Modernisation Agency supports NHS clinicians and managers in their efforts to deliver improvements to their services. The best-performing organisations stand to gain more power to make decisions locally. The Agency also supports NHS organisations whose services are poor or failing, by identifying problems and helping to get these organisations back on track.

FASCINATING FACT

Special Health Authorities are health authorities which provide a health service to the whole of England, not just to a local community. An example is the National Blood Authority.

NHS WALK-IN CENTRES

The first NHS Walk-in Centres opened in January 2000. These centres offer fast access to health advice and treatment. They are open and available to anyone and provide:

- a seven-days-a-week service, from early in the morning until late in the evening
- assessment by an experienced NHS nurse
- treatment for minor injuries and illnesses
- instant access to health advice and information on other local services
- advice on how to stay healthy
- information on local out-of-hours GP and dental services
- information on local pharmacy services.

NHS DIRECT
NHS Direct is a 24-hour phone line, staffed by nurses, which offers instant access to healthcare advice. NHS Direct nurses provide advice and support on self-treatment or pass the caller on to the appropriate service. If a serious condition or an emergency is reported, the nurse will give speedy advice on what to do, and may call an ambulance. You can find information and advice about the most common illnesses, and a range of treatments for them, on NHS Direct online or by phoning NHS Direct on 0845 4647. NOTE: In April 2004, NHS Direct became a Special Health Authority.

CARE TRUSTS

Care Trusts are organisations that work in both health and social care. They may carry out a range of services, including social care, mental health services or primary care services. Care Trusts are set up when the NHS and Local Authorities agree to work closely together, usually when a closer relationship between health and social care is needed or would benefit local care services. The number of Care Trusts is set to increase in the future.

SECONDARY CARE

If a health problem cannot be sorted out through primary care, or there is an emergency, the next stop is hospital. If you need hospital treatment, a GP will normally arrange it for you. NHS hospitals provide acute and specialist services, treating conditions that normally cannot be dealt with by primary care specialists. Primary Care Trusts are responsible for planning secondary care. They look at the health needs of the local community and develop plans to improve health and set priorities locally. They then decide which secondary care services to commission to meet people's needs. Therefore they work closely with the providers of the secondary care services that they commission to agree about delivering those services.

MENTAL HEALTH SERVICES

These can be provided through your GP, other primary care services, or through more specialist care. This might include counselling and other psychological therapies, community and family support, or general health screening. For example, people suffering bereavement, depression, stress or anxiety can get help from primary care or informal community support, or they may be referred for specialist care. Specialist care is normally provided by specialist mental health services in NHS hospital trusts or local council social services departments. Services range from psychological therapy, through to very specialist medical and training services for people with severe mental health problems.

HEALTH PROMOTION ENGLAND (HPE)

HPE was established in April 2000 following the closure of the Health Education Authority. It develops and delivers public education campaigns and promotes healthy living by focusing in particular on:

- alcohol
- children and families
- drugs
- immunisation
- older people
- sexual health.

It works in partnership with national and local organisations, both statutory and voluntary, to provide support to health and other professionals at local and community level. It is part of the NHS and works under contract to the Department of Health and the Department of Trade and Industry.

GPs

GPs look after the health of people in their local community and deal with a whole range of health problems. They also provide health education and advice on things like smoking and diet, run clinics, give vaccinations and carry out simple surgical operations. GPs usually work with a team including nurses, health visitors and midwives, as well as other health professionals such as physiotherapists and occupational therapists. If a GP cannot deal with your problem themselves, they'll usually refer you to a hospital for tests, treatment or to see a consultant with specialised knowledge. Every UK citizen has a right to be registered with a local GP, and visits to the surgery are free.

The Department of Health has set out its Improvement, Expansion and Reform Plan for 2003–6. Here is an extract from it:
'The NHS plans, to deliver an increase in the range and quality of services, and improve the service user's experience. During these three years the whole health and social care system will be changing with most notably:

- more choice for patients
- payment being made for results in the NHS so increasing the incentive for delivery
- new incentives for both social services and health to provide appropriate services for older people outside hospital
- increasing freedom for high performing organisations, including the establishment of the first foundation hospitals in the NHS.

'The health and social care priorities are:

- improving access to all services through:
- – better emergency care
- – reduced waiting, increased booking for appointments and admission and more choice for patients
- focusing on improving services and outcomes in:
- – cancer
- – coronary heart disease
- – mental health
- – older people
- – improving life chances for children
- improving the overall experience of patients
- reducing health inequalities
- contributing to the cross-government drive to reduce drug misuse.

> 'There will be the new National Service Frameworks for children and renal services and the delivery of that for diabetes.
>
> 'In order to deliver in the priority areas it will be necessary in most cases to have additional capacity available in terms of staff, facilities and equipment. In some cases this may mean involving new organisations in providing services and care.'

SALARIES FOR NURSING AND MIDWIFERY IN THE NHS

Most hospitals now employ nurses on a contract that includes internal rotation, whereby the staff rotate their shifts from day duty to night duty to give the ward 24-hours-a-day cover with the correct skill mix (a mixture of different grades of staff, outlined below). The day shifts are divided up into either early/late shifts, or long days, which can involve a 12- or 14-hour day. Different wards, hospitals and NHS Trusts employ different shift patterns, and you should take account of this when job hunting.

> On 1 April 2004, national salary scales for nurses, midwives and health visitors were increased by 3.225 per cent.

Grade A (Age 18+) Auxiliary & Assistants. From £10,375 to £13,025.
Untrained nurses, known as healthcare assistants or auxiliaries. Grade A nurses carry out many of the practical functions of ward work and the job entails a lot of hands-on nursing care.

Grade B Auxiliary & Assistants. From £12,210 to £14,370.
Also untrained and known as healthcare assistants or auxiliaries, Grade B nurses usually either have many years' experience or have completed a National Vocational Qualifications (NVQ) course in care.

Grade C Enrolled & Auxiliary. From £13,900 to £17,060.
Some grade C nurses are qualified to enrolled level.

Grade D Newly Qualified Nurses. From £17,060 to £18,830.
Grade D is either for enrolled nurses or is the grade at which a newly qualified, registered nurse starts.

Grade E Experienced Staff Nurse (Midwives normally start at this grade). From £18,230 to £22,015.
A grade E nurse has usually had at least six months' post-registration experience, and more often a full year. Many specialities such as Intensive Care Units (ITUs) or Accident and Emergency (A&E) will train their E grade nurses in the speciality they have chosen. Nurses specialise by undertaking post-registration courses. Grade E nurses should be encouraged to gain management experience, with supervision and guidance from senior nurses.

Grade F Senior Nurse. From £20,220 to £25,250.
Grade F Senior Nurse. From £25,710 to £26,180.
Grade F nurses are known as senior staff nurse or junior sister. They usually have one or two post-registration courses and have specialised in a particular area of nursing. A grade F nurse will have a considerable management role to play, and in a ward setting may be left in charge on a regular basis.

Grade G Sister/Charge Nurse (Health Visitors normally start at this grade). From £23,860 to £28,070.
Grade G Senior/Charge Nurse. From £28,550 to £29,035.
Grade G nurses are sisters or charge nurses. They are usually responsible for an entire ward or unit and all the staff. They have a considerable management role to play, which may involve more paperwork than hands-on nursing, though this varies between specialities.

Grade H Nurse Specialist. From £26,650 to £30,975.
Grade H Nurse Specialist. From £31,465 to £31,960.
Grade H Modern Matron. From £26,650 to £31,960.
Nurses who have reached this grade are usually in a management position, which involves personnel management, as well as budgeting, recruitment and training.

Grade I Nurse Specialist. From £29,515 to £33,920.
Grade I Nurse Specialist. From £34,420 to £34,920.
Grade I Modern Matron. From £29,515 to £34,920.
This grade is personnel management, decision-making, planning and policy.

Nurse/Midwife/Health Visitor Consultants. From £36,165 to £49,740.

Please note – information on pay and allowances can be found on the Department of Health website: www.doh.gov.uk/coinh.html.

RECORD GROWTH OF NHS WORKFORCE — March 2004

More NHS staff are reducing deaths, speeding up treatment and improving choice for patients than ever before, according to the latest annual NHS workforce census. This follows a record increase in the number of nurses, GPs and consultants working in the NHS.

Latest figures show that there are now 1,282,900 people working in the NHS – including 386,400 nurses, 109,000 doctors and 122,100 scientists and therapists. In 2003 alone the NHS workforce expanded by 18,800 more nurses, 5,600 more doctors and 2,500 more allied health professionals. Of the total workforce, 84 per cent are directly involved in patient care while managers and senior managers make up only 3 per cent.

Health secretary John Reid said: 'This census shows that the NHS has more doctors, nurses, scientists and therapists than ever before – as we promised in *The NHS Plan*. The whole purpose of increasing staff numbers is to deliver better patient care. The whole NHS team – Britain's biggest army for good – play their part. Providing care in new and better ways, they have helped reduce cancer deaths for under 75-year-olds by 10 per cent and deaths from coronary heart disease by 23 per cent over the last few years.

'Despite the record increases in the numbers of doctors and nurses this year, I know the NHS still struggles with shortages in some specialities and we all have a lot more to do.

'I can't create skilled medical professionals overnight but the Government is putting in place the training places needed for the future – for instance, in opening four new medical schools this year. That's why I am delighted that we have a record number of medical students training to become the next generation of NHS doctors.'

NHS chief executive Sir Nigel Crisp said: 'This increase in staffing is very encouraging. It is the people in the NHS who are responsible for the real changes we are seeing in patient care, the falling waiting times, the improvements in mortality and survival rates, cancer and coronary heart disease – in fact the progress we see now everywhere in the NHS.'

More at www.publications.doh.gov.uk/public/work_workforce.htm

GOING PRIVATE

Another option is to do private sector nursing and midwifery.

If you work in this sector as a nurse, you could find yourself working:

- for a consultant
- in a private clinic
- in a private hospital
- in a private nursing home
- in people's homes
- in a private residential home
- on a cruise ship
- in a hotel
- on a health farm
- in a private children's home
- in a private convalescent home
- with cosmetic surgery patients

- with abortion services
- with industry/commerce
- in a boarding school
- in a specialist fertility clinic
- with a pharmaceutical company
- with air ambulance services.

As a midwife in the private sector, you could work in a private clinic or nursing home or in people's homes.

SALARIES FOR PRIVATE NURSING AND MIDWIFERY

As a private nurse, you may be paid either by a nursing agency which sends you out on various assignments (you could be working in an NHS hospital), or direct by the patient if you are employed by them or via the hospital or clinic you work for. You can find temporary, permanent and contract nursing work via agencies that pay between £10 and £25 per hour. Here are some examples of how much you could earn as a private nurse in central London:

- Nurse Advisor for asthma, £15 per hour
- GP Liaison Nurse, £25,000 per year

Most independent midwives charge around £2,000–£2,500 for seeing women through their pregnancy and labour. Midwives are as flexible as they can afford to be, and can often arrange for staged payments over a period of time.

So there we have it – do you fancy being an NHS nurse or midwife or do you want to go private? Or how about working for the armed forces? Read on to find out how you can travel the world and still empty bedpans.

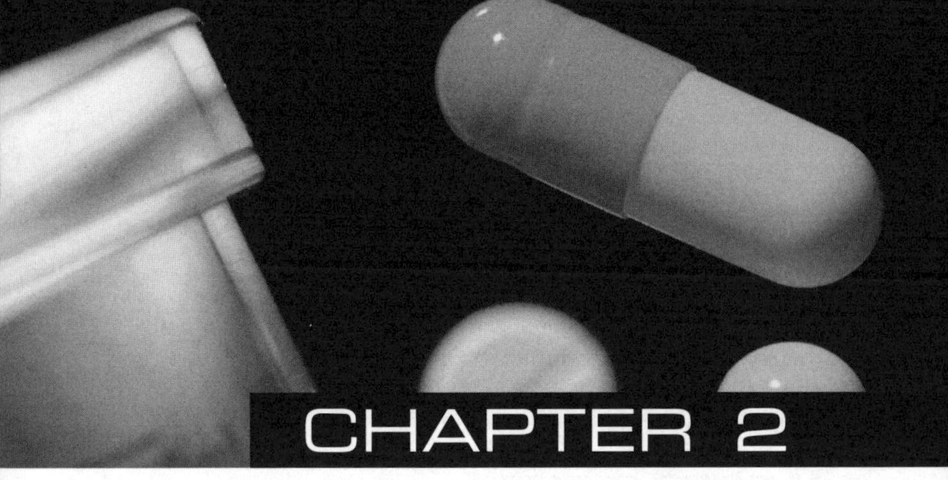

Working for the Armed Forces

The NHS or private healthcare isn't the only option you have. How about being a nurse in the Army, Navy or Air Force and seeing the world?

ARMY

Army nurses (Queen Alexandra's Royal Army Nursing Corps (QARANQ) – the QAs) are based in medical centres where they work with Army GPs or perhaps on the ward.

There are hospitals and medical centres in Cyprus, Canada, the Falkland Islands and Germany as well as the UK. Some nurses also travel to New Zealand, Australia, Kenya or South Africa, for example. There are nurses and healthcare assistants currently working in field hospitals and with medical regiments in Bosnia, Kosovo, Afghanistan and Iraq and they have also been involved in humanitarian work in Rwanda and Angola.

Army nurses have the opportunity to work in a variety of different areas away from hospitals and medical centres. This could be in military training, with Territorial Army units, with a medical regiment, field hospital or nurse education.

You start your Army career with approximately three months' military training, learning the skills you need as an officer or soldier. Qualified nurses have the opportunity to specialise, for example in A&E, intensive care or theatre.

NURSING OFFICER

As part of the multidisciplinary team you take an active role in the professional and personal development of the junior members of your nursing team including student nurses and healthcare assistants. You assist the ward manager with the day-to-day running of the ward and deputise in their absence. Because you are taking on the role of a junior ward sister/charge nurse you need to have at least two years' experience as a registered nurse (Adult or Mental Health).

You attend the ten-week entry officers' course with four weeks at the Royal Military Academy, Sandhurst. When you complete your initial training you start work in a hospital unit in the UK.

You will have access to a wide variety of fully funded study days and the opportunity after one year to apply for one of a range of post-registration courses. This could be a specialist course such as A&E/ITU or the Diploma or BSc (Hons) in Military Nursing Studies.

> FASCINATING FACT
>
> **Registered nurses who succeed in commissioning may be eligible for a bonus of £8,000 if they hold a qualification in ITU or A&E nursing.**

Depending on your previous full-time experience you will start as either a Lieutenant or Captain. When you have sufficient experience you can go on to train as a Regimental Nursing Officer, work with a medical regiment or field hospital or move into a non-nursing role such as training newly commissioned officers. Nursing officers have the potential to reach the rank of Colonel.

REGISTERED NURSE (ADULT)

As a registered adult nurse you will work in modern, busy hospitals with the highest standards of care. When you first join, you go to the Army Training Regiment at Winchester for 12 weeks' initial training as a soldier.

If you are newly qualified you start work on the wards with a period of preceptorship. You will have access to a wide variety of fully funded study days and the opportunity after one year to apply for one of a wide range of post-registration courses. This could be, for example, a specialist course within your area of interest or the Diploma or BSc (Hons) in Military Nursing Studies.

When you complete basic training and start work on the wards you will be promoted by two ranks to Acting Corporal. Further promotion is then based on ability and experience. After two years you are eligible to apply for a commission and, if successful, you will take on the additional responsibilities of a nursing officer.

Registered nurses with either the ITU or A&E qualification may be eligible for a bonus of £8,000 upon entry into the Corps. Salary on qualification is £22,549.

REGISTERED NURSE (MENTAL HEALTH)

As a registered mental health nurse you will bring your unique skills to the multidisciplinary team caring for military patients in the community, in hospitals and on operations worldwide.

Post-traumatic stress disorder, alcohol abuse and occupational psychiatry are particular specialities and the work is all acute.

When you first join you go to the Army Training Regiment at Winchester for 12 weeks' initial training as a soldier. When you complete your initial training you are likely to start work in a hospital unit in the UK, but it may not be long before you are overseas.

You start work on the wards with a period of preceptorship. You will have access to a wide variety of fully funded study days and the opportunity after one year to apply for a post-registration course on a full-time, part-time or open learning basis.

When you complete basic training and start work on the wards you will be promoted by two ranks to Acting Corporal. Further promotion is then based on ability and experience. After two years you are eligible to apply for a commission and, if successful, you will take on the additional responsibilities of a nursing officer. Salary on qualification is £22,549.

If you decide to leave, your experience in the army and any additional qualifications you gain will be highly sought after within both the NHS and the private sector.

STUDENT NURSE

This is a three-year university course to qualify as a registered nurse with a Diploma of Higher Education. Both the adult and mental health branches are available. You need to have five academic GCSEs grade C and above including English, a science subject and preferably Maths. There are a number of acceptable alternatives, for example NVQ Level 3 (Advanced) or a BTEC National Certificate or Diploma. NVQs and BTECs must be in a health-related subject.

Students who have commenced, or intend to commence, nurse training with a civilian university may be eligible for sponsorship. If you are interested in soldier entry you may receive a bursary of £5,000 over the period of your training. Upon qualification you will attend recruit training and upon completion will commence your staff nurse career as an Acting Corporal with a wage in excess of £22,000.

Candidates who wish to pursue a career as an officer may receive a bursary of £6,000 during their time in university. Upon qualification and completion of the Entry Officer Course you will be commissioned as a 2nd Lieutenant in the QARANC (but you will be paid as a Lieutenant – current salary is over £24,000).

When you first start you will join other student nurses at the Army Training Regiment in Winchester for your basic military training. This is followed by an orientation week also including Navy and RAF student nurses. You then start your training at the university. You will gain most of your practical experience in a variety of military hospital units and civilian hospitals.

Your salary during initial three-month military training is £11,121. Phase 2 salary, e.g. whilst at university, is from £13,045 rising to £16,549.

'I joined the Army to train as a nurse in 1988. I chose the Army for the variety of opportunity and because of its excellent reputation for training high-calibre nurses. I trained as a registered nurse and went on to do the Diploma in A&E Nursing among many other professional courses. I was commissioned as a nursing officer in 1994 in the rank of Lieutenant. My military career so far has taken me to many postings in this country and overseas. Most recently I worked with a field hospital, which included an operational tour to Bosnia. In Bosnia I was the Senior Nursing Officer at the British field hospital in Sipovo. Our unit was responsible for all the NATO troops in our area, and the emergency healthcare for the local civilian population.

'I commanded the nursing troop, which consisted of 13 nurses. Our responsibilities included running an 18-bed ward, the outpatients clinic and providing an on-call Intensive Treatment and Resuscitation facility. From the outset it was clear that there were not enough of us to deal with the workload, so we began an intensive training

> **programme to ensure that we could all work together as a team in any of the clinical areas as the need arose. Flexibility and teamwork always makes the difference and we were able to deal with all the challenges the hospital faced.'**
>
> **Army student nurse to Army nursing officer**

MEDICAL SERVICES TERRITORIAL ARMY

Nurses can work as trained volunteers in the Medical Services Territorial Army. There is usually a required commitment to attend at least 19 training days per year, consisting of 15 days' annual camp and two weekends. Training includes battlefield trauma life support and understanding the primary medical care needs of soldiers in the field. Military training involves physical exercise and basic level weapons training, e.g. to enable you to unload an injured soldier's rifle in the field. Training exercises take place in specialist units such as field hospitals and specially converted medical trains, which can be deployed worldwide. The role also involves teaching a wide range of TA personnel with and without medical backgrounds.

The Army's Online Careers Team: www.army.mod.uk/careers

NAVY

NURSING OFFICER

As an officer in Queen Alexandra's Royal Naval Nursing Service (QARNNS), you will be caring for service and civilian personnel. You will have the opportunity to move periodically between clinical areas or to primary care with no loss of seniority or grading.

As in an NHS hospital, you will have staff nurses and other healthcare professionals working with you, and nursing students to train in accordance with the UKCC syllabus. QARNNS is committed to the concept of Project 2000 and you will be involved in teaching nursing students undertaking the clinical component of their three-year course. You will also play an important role in teaching probationary medical assistants.

QARNNS personnel do not serve at sea in their normal peacetime role but do have a liability for Sea Service in times of tension or war and could be called upon to serve in a hospital ship or in a medical team attached to a warship.

As a nursing officer you will be responsible for a group of your staff known in the Navy as a Division, who will look to you not only for their professional welfare and development but also for help and advice on any personal or family problem they may have.

A commission as a nursing officer in QARNNS is open to registered general nurses, men and women, who are under 39 years of age and have at least two years' post-registration general experience in a busy hospital. A further professional qualification is an advantage.

All nursing officers join the Service initially on a five-year Short Career Commission. You have the option to apply to extend to eight years. During the period of your Short Career Commission you have the opportunity to apply for a Medium Career Commission (16 years) and subsequently to apply for a Full Career Commission, both of which are pensionable.

You will join in the rank of Sub-Lieutenant or Lieutenant depending on your post-qualification experience. If you begin as a Sub-Lieutenant you can normally expect to become a Lieutenant within two years. Promotion to more senior rank is by selection.

NAVAL NURSING

QARNNS is responsible for the health and fitness of all who belong to the Royal Navy and Royal Marines. QARNNS nurses, male and female, work in hospitals and also in Naval medical centres in a variety of shore establishments throughout the country. There are also limited opportunities for service overseas.

To join QARNNS as a student nurse you have to be aged between 17½ and 33. You will need to have a minimum of five GCSEs at grade C or equivalent in academic subjects, which must include English language plus either Maths or a science subject, or a BTEC National Diploma or a GNVQ Advanced level or equivalent.

To join as a staff nurse you have to be aged between 21 and 33 and a RGN/RN on Part 1, 12, 13 or 15 of the UKCC Register, and recently qualified or lacking the experience to fill a junior ward sister/charge nurse post. All QARNNS ratings begin their naval career at HMS *Raleigh*. As well as learning the basics of marching, wearing your uniform, naval traditions and history, you will be trained in firefighting and security. You will also learn team skills in exercises on Dartmoor. Once you have completed the eight weeks' Naval General Training you will start your professional training.

Royal Naval Nursing Service Reserve

The Queen Alexandra's Royal Naval Nursing Service Reserve (QARNNS)(R) allows nurses to contribute to the QARNNS on a voluntary basis. Members of the QARNNS(R) undertake a minimum of 12 days' Operational Role Training per year, which includes learning to man Primary Casualty Receiving Ships in crisis and war. There is also a requirement to attend a number of drill nights and to be available for some weekends.

Reserves are also liable to compulsory call-out in a national emergency or in support of military operations and disaster relief.

After initial training at HMS *Raleigh* you will spend two weeks on a Nurse Orientation Course at the Health Studies Division of the Royal Defence Medical College. You then commence training for your Diploma, which takes three years. During part of the university summer vacation, you will undertake a further period of naval general training, which involves leadership, management and a variety of physical activities to maintain personal fitness. Naval nurses follow the syllabus set by the English National Board. The first 18 months of your training will be on the Common Foundation programme and will be based at the University of Portsmouth and RH Haslar with colleagues from the other two services.

The second 18 months will be adult branch training. Specialist experience in psychiatry, obstetrics, care of the elderly and community nursing takes place in civilian district hospitals and the community. On completion of training, a graduation ceremony is held at the university for the award of your Diploma of Higher Education and Registered Nurse Qualification. Following UKCC registration and the PBPQC, naval nurses may be drafted to RH Haslar for post-registration experience before being drafted elsewhere in the Royal Navy.

During your career, there may be the opportunity to undertake post-basic nursing courses to specialise in a particular area such as intensive care or A&E nursing. Generally you will need to have been in the Service for a minimum of two years before applying, and there may be a return of service depending on the length of the course. Two years after registration it may be possible for you to be considered for a commission as a nursing officer (ward sister) providing you reach the necessary standards, are recommended and are successful at the Admiralty Interview Board. For those who do not wish to consider a commission, the naval career structure enables you to progress to Warrant Officer, the highest non-commissioned rate available to naval nurses.

Royal Navy or Royal Marines career enquiries, tel: 0845 607 5555

AIR FORCE

NURSING OFFICER

A career in the Princess Mary's Royal Air Force Nursing Service (PMRAFNS) offers variety. You could be working on a ward in Cyprus, in a specialist unit in the UK, or even 30,000 feet up in a Tristar on aeromedical evacuation duties.

You are encouraged to take English National Board (ENB) courses relevant to Service needs, and pursue your professional training in line with the Post-Registration Education and Practice of the UK Central Council. To this end, the RAF will allow you study time and pay your fees.

Age:	23–38
Pay:	£24,181–£70,300
Rank:	Officer
Minimum length of service:	Six years
Qualifications:	Professional. GCSE/CSEs must include English language and maths.

STAFF NURSE (REGISTERED MENTAL NURSE)

As a staff nurse (RMN) you'll work in a team with people from many different disciplines, including psychiatry, at departments of community psychiatry. In undertaking your duties, you'll know and understand the specialised diagnostic procedures and modern treatments using drug therapy, social skills and individual psychotherapy necessary for psychiatric nursing care. Following additional training, staff nurses (RMN) may be employed on the Aeromedical Evacuation Squadron based at RAF Lyneham. There, it will be your responsibility to provide psychiatric nursing care to those service personnel and dependants requiring repatriation and aeromedical evacuation to the UK.

Age:	21–32
Pay:	£22,550–£38,300
Rank:	Trade
Minimum length of service:	Nine years
Qualifications:	Professional – RMN/NMC

STAFF NURSE (REGISTERED GENERAL NURSE)

The PMRAFNS helps looks after the health and fitness of everyone in the RAF, whether they're aircrew, groundcrew or other support staff. PMRAFNS nurses also provide care for entitled civilians and personnel from other services.

Age:	21–32
Pay:	£22,550–£38,300
Rank:	Trade
Minimum length of service:	Nine years
Qualifications:	Professional – RGN/NMC

STUDENT STAFF NURSE

The PMRAFNS offers a three-year training course for student nurses within the Faculty of Health and Community Care at the University of Central England. About half your time is spent on clinical placements, which take place at both NHS and military establishments. Successful graduation will lead to registration as a registered nurse (adult) on the Professional Register of the Nursing and Midwifery Council (NMC, see page 105 for details) together with the award of a Diploma of Higher Education or a BSc (Honours) in Nursing. You'll then enter productive service as a staff nurse (RGN).

Age:	17½–32
Pay:	Up to £14,991
Rank:	Trade
Minimum length of service:	Nine years
Qualifications:	Five GCSEs/SCEs at grade C/3 minimum or equivalent to include English language, Maths and a science-based subject

For more information, contact the Nursing Liaison Team on 01400 261201, ext 6782, or email nslo@raf-careers.raf.mod.uk.

Not sure whether you want to travel the world? Want to find out more about the wide variety of nursing opportunities in general? Read on.

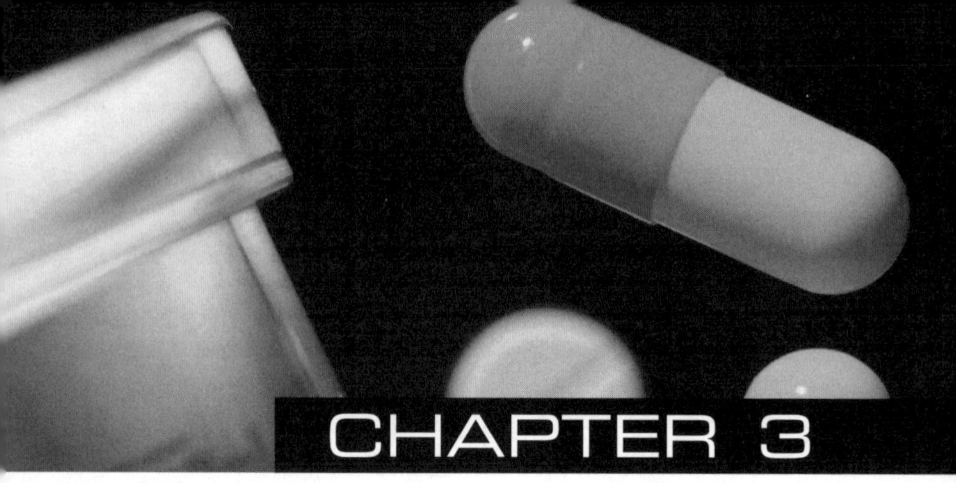

Where nursing could take you

ACCIDENT AND EMERGENCY NURSING (A&E)

'Nurses working in the accident and emergency setting initiate the immediate care of patients with undifferentiated and undiagnosed problems, decide upon the priorities for care and prescribe, initiate and monitor interventions...'

The RCN (Royal College of Nursing) Faculty of Emergency Nursing

A&E nurses:

- receive and resuscitate seriously ill patients
- give expert advice (via the telephone or face-to-face)
- provide support to the bereaved

- deal with child-abuse issues
- teach student nurses, nurse learners and medical staff new to the department.

Depending on the A&E nurse's level of expertise, they will also take responsibility for leading a team, working without supervision and setting priorities within the A&E service.

BLOOD TRANSFUSION NURSING

Blood transfusion nurses assess the health and fitness of potential donors and support them through the blood donation process. There are three main types of collection teams:

- Mobile blood collection teams.
- Apheresis donor suites linked to blood centres. During the donation process the blood is separated out, some components are removed and those that aren't needed are returned to the donor.
- Static donor centres in inner cities.

The main responsibilities include: caring for, counselling and undertaking health checks on voluntary donors, undertaking venepuncture, staff training, monitoring, assessment and clinical supervision, supporting unregistered care staff (known as donor carers) and undertaking research and audit. Blood transfusion nurses also support a range of patient-linked or therapeutic services, such as stem cell harvesting and plasma exchange regimes.

BREAST CARE NURSING

There are around 400 breast care nurses working in the UK. Breast care nurses provide information, care and support to women who have, or fear they may have, breast cancer. Breast care nurses:

- provide counselling
- work with the multidisciplinary team, including physiotherapists, prosthetic fitting services, social workers and psychiatrists
- offer advice and guidance on suitable bras and swimwear. Some breast care nurses run their own prosthetic fitting service
- provide breast awareness education to targeted groups in the community
- educate nurses, medical and other staff on the psychological care of patients with breast cancer
- run self-help groups.

CHILDREN'S NURSING

Children react to illness in a very different way to adults, and need to be cared for and supported by specially trained nurses who understand their particular needs. Those qualified in the children's branch of nursing work with 0- to 18-year-olds in a variety of settings, from specialist baby care units to adolescent services. Once qualified, it is possible to specialise in areas such as burns and plastics, intensive care, child protection and cancer care.

Children's nurses work closely with patients' families as part of the caring process. The job is to give the child's carers the confidence and ability to carry on with their caring role, knowing when to stand back and when to take over if necessary.

Within the community there are opportunities to work as a community children's nurse, a practice nurse or a clinical nurse specialist, working with children with complex health needs such as diabetes and cystic fibrosis. Children's nurses also work for the school nursing service. In the acute sector, children's nurses work on generalist and specialist in-patient wards, as well as in outpatients, intensive care and day care services. A&E departments employ children's nurses, as approximately one-third of attendees at A&E departments are children. Children's nurses liaise with various agencies, including those working for social services and the police. Some hospitals have a specialist adolescent unit, and many maternity units include a neonatal intensive care unit that employs children's nurses.

In the independent sector there are a number of posts for children's nurses in private hospitals. Many independent schools, particularly residential and boarding schools, employ a school nurse or matron.

CHILD PROTECTION NURSING

Broadly the role of the child protection nurse involves working with children on a one-to-one basis, with families, communities, self-help groups and pressure groups. It also involves teamwork with other agencies to help children to maintain their human rights. Each strategic health authority in England and Wales has a designated nurse who takes the lead, along with a designated doctor, on child protection issues across all services. The designated nurse may be employed by a specific trust, but works across service boundaries. The role involves:

- acting as an important source of advice
- promoting and influencing relevant training
- representing local health services on the area child protection committee.

MARIE CURIE NURSE OF THE YEAR

Catherine Le Roy was named Marie Curie Nurse of the Year for England at a ceremony hosted by Prince Charles at St James's Palace. Catherine, 39, who works as a community nurse in Bristol, was chosen from more than 3,000 fellow nurses after being nominated by colleagues, managers and patients. Prince Charles, who is president of Marie Curie Cancer Care, wished Catherine and her colleagues well, saying: 'The presence of a Marie Curie

nurse in the home makes a tremendous difference to both patients and their carers.'

Catherine has been a nurse for 18 years, qualifying at Guy's Hospital in 1983 and joining Marie Curie just over two years ago to provide out-of-hours care to home-based patients. For the next year Catherine will be helping to raise the profile of the Marie Curie charity, while still working as a nurse.

'I'm just delighted to have the opportunity to raise awareness of the work of Marie Curie Cancer Care and generate support for the charity', she said.

June 2001

CONSULTANT POSTS – NURSE, MIDWIFE AND HEALTH VISITOR

These new post holders spend a minimum of 50 per cent of their time working directly with patients, ensuring that people using the NHS continue to benefit from the very best nursing and midwifery skills. In addition, the new nurse consultants are responsible for developing personal practice, being involved in research and evaluation and contributing to education, training and development.

DAY SURGERY NURSING

Nurses working in day surgery units assess, plan, deliver and evaluate the care of patients undergoing a range of surgical procedures, including ear, nose and throat, oral, urology, plastic and cosmetic surgery, cataract removal, endoscopy, orthopaedic and pain-relieving procedures. Day surgery nurses manage the patient's whole episode of care, from admission, assessment and preparation for surgery, to monitoring and recovery after surgery and discharge management. Some units are attached to a theatre suite.

NURSING ON EXPEDITIONS AND HOLIDAYS
The main aim of the role of expedition nurse is usually to assist in the adequate preparation of expedition members in respect of appropriate advice and information on health issues before departure and to help maintain the health and welfare of the expedition members whilst overseas. Nursing on an expedition necessitates a sound knowledge of first aid, and expedition organisations often look for experience in A&E. Tropical disease experience or completion of a relevant course may also be useful. Contracts are usually for short periods only, varying from a couple of weeks to several months.

DERMATOLOGY NURSING

Dermatology nursing is practised in community, general practice and acute settings, by those employed as tissue viability nurses, nurse practitioners or specialist nurses. The dermatology nurse role includes:

- treating acute and complex dermatological conditions
- patch-testing people with allergy problems
- helping teenagers deal with acne
- helping clients come to terms with the psychological, social and physical consequences of their condition
- teaching clients to use make-up or wigs as camouflage
- involvement with clinical trials and audit
- teaching other healthcare professionals.

Many dermatology nurses run their own clinics, where they are involved with a range of activities such as removal of warts, port wine stains or tattoos, assessing and treating leg ulcers, running ultraviolet light treatments or undertaking laser procedures.

CASE STUDY

THE MOTOR NEURONE DISEASE SPECIALIST

Ruth qualified at the Royal Free Hospital in 1991 as a registered nurse, and worked in oncology and neurosurgery before finally choosing to specialise in the area of neurology. Over the years she backpacked her way around the world with friends, gaining experience working as a nurse in Australia, and eventually returning home to settle in England. Whilst in Australia she became involved in the initiation of a new scheme for the care of people with MND (motor neurone disease) and their loved ones. Ruth started working as a clinical nurse specialist for a MND multidisciplinary clinic, which aimed to improve the quality of life for patients with MND via an outpatient clinic, and she co-ordinated this from its conception in September 1999 to December 2000, when she returned to England.

The challenges of this job were wide and varied, including teaching staff, liaising with internal and external health professionals, fundraising, presenting at conferences, improving awareness in the community, implementing patient/carer/staff questionnaires to review service and, most importantly, providing a link between people with MND, their carers and the multidisciplinary team. The clinic involved all members of the multidisciplinary team, a neurologist, a thoracic physician, the MND Association of New South Wales, a nurse consultant in respiratory medicine, a nurse specialist in MND and Ruth. The main emphasis of the clinic was teamwork, to ensure excellent communication between all the above-mentioned, the person affected with MND and his/her loved ones.

When Ruth returned to England her aim was to stay within the speciality of MND and so she became involved with the vital research and support service being offered at Charing Cross Hospital.

DISTRICT/COMMUNITY NURSING

Working in partnership with patients and their carers in the community, district and community nurses assess healthcare needs and develop appropriate packages of care. They are often based in GP surgeries.

FAMILY PLANNING NURSING

Family planning nurses work in GP practices, sexual health clinics, women's health centres, teenage clinics and abortion services. Many nurses who provide family planning advice and care are employed as practice nurses. Family planning nurses provide some or all of the following services:

- contraceptive and sexual health advice
- clinical assessment and care
- cervical screening
- sexual health education and breast awareness.

Many specialist family planning services have had funding withdrawn, and consequently practice nurses who are family planning trained are increasingly undertaking this role.

FERTILITY NURSING

Fertility nurses work in hospital settings, primary care and the independent sector, in specialist fertility clinics or departments. A typical role includes the following:

- counselling, educating and supporting couples undergoing fertility treatment
- co-ordinating investigations such as blood tests, semen analysis, tests for tubal patency and imaging uterine cavities
- performing procedures such as ultrasound, guided oocyte retrieval and percutaneous epididymal sperm aspiration
- running nurse-led clinics
- co-ordinating the work of treatment centres, including business planning and budget management.

GYNAECOLOGY NURSING

Gynaecology nurses assess, plan, implement and evaluate the care of women before and after gynaecological surgery. They provide counselling and support to help alleviate patients' anxiety, and give health advice. Teaching, providing information and counselling clients undergoing surgery is an important part of the role. Some nurses run pre-admission clinics.

HAEMOPHILIA NURSING

Haemophilia nurses plan, deliver and evaluate care given to patients with haemophilia in hospital. This requires competence in venepuncture and cannulation for treatment administration and blood sampling. In some haemophilia centres, nurses review and treat patients autonomously, according to group protocols. Very few patients now require hospitalisation, so specialist nurses act as a vital link between hospital and home, where patients and carers are taught how to administer treatment.

HEALTH VISITOR

Health visitors carry out developmental screening of children and provide health education programmes for individuals and communities. Some work from doctors' surgeries while others cover a geographical area, visiting people in their homes and schools. Health visitors work with a large network of other groups concerned with health, sickness, social and educational services. As a key member of the primary healthcare team, it's the health visitor's job to promote health in the practice area (most health visitors cover the area of a GP's practice). They help well people to stay well, and ill people to come to terms with their illness. A health visitor could be counselling the previous partners of someone diagnosed HIV positive, paying visits to mothers who have postnatal depression, or supporting and advising someone who wants to give up smoking.

Health visitors must be qualified nurses. They then take a degree programme to qualify as a health visitor.

IN-FLIGHT NURSING

In-flight nurses assist with the repatriation of patients with a variety of illnesses in scheduled or dedicated aircraft or air ambulances. Common conditions include stroke, heart attack, angina, pneumonia, orthopaedic problems, respiratory difficulties, burns and multiple trauma. Patients include neonates and those with mental health problems. The role includes:

- initial health assessment
- obtaining tickets
- caring for patients during their flight, often through phone communication with medical staff
- ensuring the safe transfer of patient property
- maintaining the safe transfer of medical equipment
- providing a door-to-door service to the patient's home or hospital.

ASHFIELD HEALTHCARE NURSE ADVISOR ROLE

Ashfield Healthcare is a major provider of contract resources to the UK and Irish pharmaceutical industries. Part of the United Drug Group, they offer a range of services including sales force resourcing, nurse advisors, vacancy management and training and development.

All nurse advisors are qualified, registered nurses, protected by and working within the guidelines of the NMC Code of Conduct and the ABPI Code of Practice. The role provides a golden opportunity to specialise in one or two particular disease areas, with increasing emphasis on promoting health improvements and helping to fulfil demanding clinical targets. Raising the standards in particular disease areas can be of huge benefit to all parties involved with a Nurse Advisor Project, which makes the role such a fulfilling one. Firstly, the surgery benefits as

they are concentrating on raising the standard of care and meeting clinical targets. More importantly, the patient benefits from the outcome and maybe a drug/therapy change, and the sponsoring pharmaceutical company gains recognition for sponsoring this additional expert resource that has helped to raise the standards of care. The nurse is in contact with many different GP practices, all with different ways of thinking, different policies and different ideas, yet all sharing the same priority of a high standard of patient care.

There are many different objectives for each project, which can include:

- data trawling
- auditing and producing detailed reports for individual surgeries
- reviewing patient therapy and recommending changes to drugs/dosages
- administering to patients
- educating both patients and health professionals within the disease therapy area
- raising the profile of the sponsoring company.

Work is carried out on a local, regional and sometimes national level, in conjunction with primary healthcare teams, pharmaceutical advisors, primary care teams and other health professionals. The work of a nurse advisor varies from day to day, week to week. The nurse advisor is responsible for filling her own diary and building up a manageable workload. This requires self-motivation and flexibility, and the results to be gained are both satisfying and rewarding.

LEARNING DISABILITY NURSING

About three per cent of the population have a learning disability. Nurses who qualify in this branch of nursing help those with learning disabilities to live independent and fulfilling lives. This may involve working with people in supported accommodation – typically three to four people with learning disabilities live together in flats or houses, with 24-hour support. Some nurses work with individuals who require more intensive support – for instance, in hospitals or in specialist secure units for offenders with learning disabilities. Others specialise in areas such as epilepsy management or working with people with sensory impairment.

The role of the nurse is to help all people with a learning disability to maintain and improve their lifestyles and to participate fully as equal members of society. This may mean helping clients to develop their manual and recognition skills so that, for instance, they can use kitchen equipment to make a pot of tea. In other cases, you will be underpinning people's efforts to find work and bring up a family – helping them make their way in a world that can sometimes seem difficult and threatening.

The emphasis is on nursing in a range of social settings, including home, work and leisure activities. You will gain experience in four main areas:

- Family settings.
- Adult education.
- Education for young people.
- Community/residential settings.

LIAISON AND DISCHARGE PLANNING NURSING

Nurses working in discharge planning lead on or help to develop effective policy and practice for the discharge of patients from hospital. This involves close liaison with primary care teams, other specialist agencies and bed management services.

MACMILLAN NURSING

The title Macmillan nurse originates through the charity Macmillan Cancer Relief, which provides funding for this specialist role. Macmillan nurses are specialists in cancer care and/or palliative care. There are four main types of Macmillan nurse:

- the home care nurse
- the hospital support nurse
- the breast care nurse
- the paediatric nurse.

Macmillan nurses work with patients and families from time of diagnosis. They provide information, control the patient's pain and symptoms and offer emotional support.

Sue Pender, a Macmillan nurse at Scarborough, Whitby and Ryedale NHS Trust, has come a long way since leaving school with two O-levels. Now, she combines the demands of Macmillan nursing with teaching district nurses about palliative care.

'After a pre-nursing course I realised that, with some hard work, I could change my future and I have.' Sue now says how fortunate she feels to have chosen a career with such diversity.

MENTAL HEALTH NURSING

Mental health nurses form therapeutic relationships with mentally ill people and their families. Their role includes helping individuals to maintain independence, to manage their condition and to overcome the stigma of mental illness. Mental health nurses are also skilled in managing challenging behaviour and defusing tense or violent situations. Mental health nurses work with GPs, psychiatrists, social workers and others to co-ordinate the care of people suffering from mental illness.

The vast majority of people with mental health problems live in the community. Nurses plan and deliver care for people living in their own home, in small residential units or specialist hospital services. Some are based in health centres. It is possible to develop expertise in areas such as rehabilitation, child and adolescent mental health, substance misuse and working with offenders. As your career develops you may choose to specialise in areas such as drugs and alcohol misuse or working with offenders. You could also become involved in education, research or management roles. Mental health nurses are also the most likely to be responsible for co-ordinating a patient's care in the community. You'll therefore find yourself liaising professionally with a wide range of other services including social workers, police, charities, local government and housing officials.

FORENSIC NURSING

Mental health nurses working in forensic settings provide care and treatment for mentally disordered offenders. The nurse is a key professional within the multidisciplinary team working to minimise the potential for dangerousness and maximise the opportunity for treatment and therapeutic regimes. Depending on their level of seniority, forensic mental health nurses:

- assess, plan, implement and evaluate nursing care for a caseload of patients in settings of medium or high security and in the community
- teach, demonstrate and supervise the practice of nursing students and unregistered nursing staff
- develop and apply evidence-based practice, maintain quality standards and take a lead in audit processes and research
- manage the ward environment
- apply risk assessment and risk management procedures

- undertake health promotion activities
- integrate security protocols with nursing practice
- provide effective clinical leadership within the multidisciplinary team.

MULTIPLE SCLEROSIS (MS) SPECIALIST NURSING

This is a relatively new role in nursing. MS specialist nurses:

- use their expert knowledge to deliver services for people ranging from those undergoing diagnostic investigations through to those with severe disability
- are skilled communicators and educators
- liaise with social/community services, primary care teams and hospitals
- have an extensive caseload of clients with MS.

NATIONAL BLOOD SERVICE

With the ongoing demand for blood, increasing commitments in tissue banking and the changing needs of the NHS, there are a variety of career opportunities in the National Blood Service. For more information, contact: National Nurse Advisor, National Blood Authority, Oak House, Reeds Crescent, Watford, Hertfordshire WD1 1QH. Tel: 01923 486800.

NURSE EDUCATIONALIST

Nurse educationalists work in the practice setting, higher education and further education. Nurse lecturers are responsible for pre- and post-registration nursing or midwifery curriculum design, teaching and assessing in higher education establishments. The role also involves undertaking research projects and providing pastoral care or individual tutorial support for students. Practice educators are responsible for teaching and development in the practice setting. They provide support and advice for all healthcare professionals, including mentors, who are involved with nursing students. They also form the link between the practice setting and higher education establishments. Further education lecturers work mainly with post-16 and/or adult learners. Nurses find employment in the further education sector through teaching on health and social care related courses including Access to Nursing/Healthcare and NVQ/SVQ programmes.

NURSERY NURSE AND PLAY SPECIALIST

For information on nursery nursing you should write to: Council for Awards in Children's Care and Education, 8 Chequer Street, St Albans, Herts AL1 3XZ. Tel: 01727 847636. Enclose SAE.

For information on a career as a play specialist you should contact: National Association of Hospital Play Staff (NAHPS), C/O Information Officer, 40 High Street, Landbeach, Cambridge CB4 8DT.

FROM NURSE TO PASTORAL CARE CO-ORDINATOR

The Diocese of Exeter has appointed its first ever Pastoral Care Co-ordinator. This is someone working half time to provide access to counselling and support services for clergy and others who work for the diocese, and their dependants. The post has been set up to respond to the increasing numbers of clergy who are suffering with stress, leading to some being off work for long periods, and a few taking early retirement on health grounds. The Co-ordinator will be Julie Barrett, who has been working near Bristol as a psychotherapist in private practice.

While working as a nurse, Julie developed her counselling skills, and then spent some time managing support services in mental health housing before going freelance. She is an active member of the Church of England, has been licensed as a Reader (authorised lay minister) since 2001, and is a member of the Franciscan Third Order. She assists in the chaplaincy of a prison. Julie, 48, has two grown-up children.

NURSING MANAGEMENT

Nursing managers work in a variety of settings. The following are examples of management roles in nursing:

- managing a ward or unit, or a group of wards and units
- managing a care home
- the modern matron role that involves providing hands-on clinical management and leadership, usually for a group of wards or units
- director or assistant director of nursing roles, where the emphasis is on nursing leadership and development
- lead nurse and team leader roles in primary care
- operational management, for which a nursing qualification is not necessarily a requirement
- executive nursing roles as a Chief Executive of a Trust, for example.

Nurses in management roles use leadership skills to, among other things, manage change, build teams, develop strategic plans, policies and procedures, lead projects, write reports, resolve conflict, give presentations, commission services, act as role models, manage resources, influence and collaborate with others and ensure practice development and quality patient/client care.

THE COMMUNITY STAFF NURSE

'My name is Helen, I'm 42 and have been a community staff nurse since 1997. I trained as a nurse following a stint of voluntary work in a local hospital and a long period of office jobs. Going back into education after leaving school at 16 seemed quite daunting, so I took a year's Access course first. These are courses designed for mature students, as an alternative to A-levels – this was an excellent preparation

for the academic side of my training. I decided to take a degree in nursing, and found some of the training quite challenging.

'There's a lot of criticism about the modern style of nurse education being too academically based with not enough hands-on practice, but the nursing role is continually changing, and the academic teaching shows you how to use research, question why decisions are made (by yourself and others) and understand the broader picture in terms of Government policies and suchlike. Practice placements can also vary greatly depending on the setting and your own particular interests. Following my elective (final) placement with a community team, I was offered a D grade post with them.

'I can honestly say I've never been bored while nursing. The first six months are a really steep learning curve, but your education continues, not only in what you learn from your personal experience but from the changes that take place in the profession. It's a unique type of job, which requires you to use a combination of learned and instinctive skills – no two situations are ever the same. Although I've always worked in the UK, there are many opportunities abroad, and nursing is a career where you can take a break and return. Overall, I'd really recommend nursing as a career – it's not like on the TV, but I've never worked in any setting that's given me so much variety and job satisfaction, and where I've met so many interesting people.'

NURSING OLDER PEOPLE

CONTINUING CARE

Nurses working in care homes, hospitals and in the client's home provide continuing care. Since April 2002 all care homes have been registered by the National Care Standards Commission. Nurses working in care homes that provide nursing services provide expert care for clients with a range of nursing needs. Increasingly, residents have similar needs to those in hospitals. Some homes specialise in caring for a particular client group, such as those with brain injury or dementia. The number of homes offering short-term intermediate and rehabilitative care has increased, following Government policy outlined in *The NHS Plan*. Nurses employed as a matron are usually responsible for the overall management of the home. In larger homes, a deputy matron or head of care is employed to manage and ensure the quality of nursing care. First and second level nurses are often in charge of a shift, which involves:

- planning, implementing and evaluating care
- mentoring, supervising and supporting healthcare assistants
- teaching and educating healthcare assistants, e.g. acting as an NVQ assessor
- organising social activities and events for the residents
- communicating with relatives and friends
- liaising with GPs and the multidisciplinary team
- ensuring that the home meets the standards set by the National Care Standards Commission.

Some care homes provide support for residents who require personal, rather than nursing, care. Personal care includes help with mobilising, hygiene and eating and drinking. Care homes that provide personal care are not required to employ registered nurses, although many homes employ a registered nurse who acts as manager or deputy manager. Many homes provide a mixture of personal and nursing care.

INTERMEDIATE CARE NURSING

The NHS Plan (England), published in 2000, included a commitment to intermediate care. Intermediate care aims to ensure that older people's contact with hospital is minimised. Nurses who co-ordinate intermediate care services help prevent older people from going into or staying in hospital. Instead, they arrange home care, a short stay in a community hospital or up to two weeks' rehabilitation in a care home. Intermediate care nurses work closely with hospitals, GPs, primary care groups/trusts, care homes and social services. They often co-ordinate rapid response teams that can prevent hospital admissions by providing care for older people in crisis in their own home. Such initiatives are often run jointly with social services. Intermediate care nurses also play a role in educating colleagues in care homes about rehabilitation and discharge planning.

OCCUPATIONAL HEALTH NURSING

Occupational health nurses work in industry, health services, commerce and education. They are employed as independent practitioners or as part of a larger occupational health service team, often attached to a personnel department. Some occupational health nurses run their own business providing occupational health advice on a consultancy basis. The occupational health nurse role includes:

- the prevention of health problems, promotion of healthy living and working conditions
- understanding the effects of work on health and health at work
- basic first aid and health screening
- workforce and workplace monitoring and health needs assessment
- health promotion
- education and training
- counselling and support
- risk assessment and risk management.

Occupational health nurses are considered to be leaders in public health in the workplace setting.

CASE STUDY

COSMETIC TREATMENT AND ANTI-HIV THERAPY

For the last ten years Odile has been working as a nurse cosmetic practitioner in Harley Street. During that time she has worked with several injectable products designed to improve physical appearance, notably in the reduction of lines and wrinkles. Many speak of their experience with lipodystrophy (changes in body shape among people taking anti-HIV therapy).

Although not life-threatening, this disease has a powerful impact on the mental well-being of the sufferer. Because the effects appear quickly, patients find themselves having to explain the change in their physical appearance to family members, friends and work colleagues who do not know their status. Most have spoken of symptoms of social withdrawal because of their condition, of giving up work, of not going to clubs, pubs or restaurants, of reducing social life and only seeing friends who know about their condition.

Some talk of knowing that 'lipodystrophic look' and associate it with the beginning of the loss of friends or loved ones through HIV-related illnesses. Most patients Odile treats are desperate for some relief from the distress of looking at themselves and knowing that they have this condition.

'The majority of patients I have treated are physically fit and well, having successfully assimilated lifestyle and diet changes in addition to complex drug regimes, and the often dramatic facial effects of lipodystrophy are the sole daily reminder of their status. Their reaction to the change in their physical appearance after treatment is overwhelmingly positive. Several clients have been offered anti-depressants to overcome their distress. Others have been offered counselling and therapy. All of these treatments cost the NHS money, and can only offer variable success rates. I feel that offering practical treatment for physical effects brings immediate quantifiable results in the well-being of sufferers.'

PAIN MANAGEMENT SPECIALIST NURSING

Nurses who specialise in pain management work in both acute and chronic pain teams. Palliative care professionals usually deal with pain caused by malignancy. Nurses who work in acute pain management play a vital role in ensuring the safe and effective treatment of acute pain caused by surgery, trauma or disease. They educate nurses and other healthcare professionals about new pain-relieving techniques, audit treatment options and may undertake research. Those involved in chronic pain management work with medical staff, physiotherapists, pharmacists, psychologists and occupational therapists to devise pain management programmes for clients. Clients usually attend a structured programme on a group basis that meets once or twice a week. Nurses play a role in monitoring the patient's use of medication and helping them to plan a drug reduction programme if that is what they wish.

PRACTICE NURSING

Practice nurses deliver care in general practice surgeries and health centres. Their role includes:

- the detection and assessment of undifferentiated needs
- involvement in the recognition of conditions such as asthma and diabetes
- management of health promotion clinics including travel health, immunisations and sexual and reproductive health
- involvement in illness prevention through screening, including breast awareness, cervical cytology and care before conception.

PRISON NURSING

The role of a prison nurse is to ensure prisoners have proper access to healthcare. Prison nurses undertake health assessment and screening and help prisoners to manage conditions such as diabetes, epilepsy, asthma and drug and alcohol dependence. Health promotion is a large part of the role. Prison nurses also care for those with mental health problems and often work with community psychiatric nurses to provide support for those at risk of self-harm, bullying, suicide and depression.

Recent reforms have led to closer partnerships with the NHS, including shared education, clinical supervision, secondment initiatives and joint specialist services. Some prison nurses are employed as civilian nurses whilst others hold a dual role, as both nurse and prison officer (often called qualified healthcare officers). In theory, those employed as qualified healthcare officers hold a more custodial role and could be required to attend riots. In practice, all those working in the prison healthcare services are required to maintain order, control and discipline, which can present a challenge for those who are new to the service.

REHABILITATION NURSING

The King's Fund defines rehabilitation as: 'a process aiming to restore personal autonomy in those aspects of daily living considered most relevant by patients or service users, and their family carers' (King's Fund (1998), *Effective practice in rehabilitation: the evidence of systematic reviews*).

Nurses who specialise in rehabilitation work in, amongst others, specialist hospital or community rehabilitation units, day care units, nurse-led clinics, continuing care and intermediate care. Some nurses work with specific clients, such as those with spinal injuries, stroke victims, those with cardiac disease or older people. The rehabilitation nurse role includes:

- drawing up rehabilitation plans based on assessment of clients' needs
- helping clients to set goals and supporting them to achieve these goals
- evaluating the effectiveness of rehabilitation plans

- taking a lead role in communicating with all relevant members of the healthcare team, family members and carers to ensure that the rehabilitation programme is effectively co-ordinated
- educating clients, relatives and other healthcare professionals about the rehabilitation process, using a variety of teaching strategies
- providing advice and counselling.

NURSE IN THE COUNTRY OF THE LONG WHITE CLOUD (or New Zealand to those of you who aren't in the know!)
New Zealand is an independent nation and a member of the British Commonwealth. It has a diverse multicultural population of around 3.8 million people. The majority of New Zealanders are of British descent, and the largest minority is New Zealand's indigenous Maori who make up around 14 per cent of the population.

Nursing work in New Zealand is similar to that in the UK. The hospitals are run by District Health Boards (DHBs), and one or more hospitals may be governed by the same DHB. The condition of the hospitals is good, and many have been upgraded in recent years. The hospitals vary in size from small 150-bed rural hospitals to large 500-bed tertiary care facilities. Most nurses work eight-hour shifts that include night duty. Many hospitals have, or are introducing, Clinical Career Pathways. The nurses working on a Career Pathway are paid according to the level they have achieved. Other nurses are paid according to their years of experience.

You need to apply for a Working Holiday Visa or Work Permit in the UK from the New Zealand High Commission; your UK Worldwide Healthcare Exchange (WHE) consultant will guide you on this.

The New Zealand Nursing Council is the registering body. Your WHE consultant will order the application form direct from the Nursing Council. Nursing Unions & Indemnity Insurance: The

New Zealand Nursing Organisation is the national union for all nursing and midwifery staff. It is not compulsory to join, but it is advisable, as you will not be covered by the collective contract if you do not. Your consultant can provide you with costs and details of how to join.

RESEARCH NURSING

Depending on their level of seniority, research nurses:

- develop, design or work towards research protocols
- play an active role in research ethical requirements, including eliciting informed consent
- identify and screen suitable patients for trials (where relevant)
- co-ordinate or undertake data collection and patient support
- enter data onto the computer
- provide data analysis
- contribute to and write reports
- provide input into local and regional research committees
- disseminate research findings
- publish papers
- submit proposals to and liaise with providers of research funding
- undertake an education and development role.

Those nurses who work in universities will often hold a combined teaching role. Research nurses are also employed in the clinical setting and by the pharmaceutical industry.

RESUSCITATION OFFICER

Resuscitation officers are responsible for the planning, organisation and implementation of resuscitation training for healthcare professionals.

RHEUMATOLOGY NURSING

Most nurses care for patients with rheumatic disease at some stage in their career. In the UK over 20 million people suffer from rheumatic conditions such as rheumatoid arthritis and metabolic bone diseases such as osteoporosis. Specialist rheumatology nurses work in the community, hospital wards, outpatient clinics, research and education. Rheumatology nurses undertake the following activities:

- assist patients and their carers to come to terms with the physical, psychological and social effects of their disease
- provide information, advice and guidance on treatment options
- run nurse-led clinics
- assess, plan, monitor, audit and evaluate care and the effects of medication
- help patients to manage their pain
- educate patients and clients about the side effects of their drugs
- liaise with and make referrals to other members of the healthcare team, such as GPs, physiotherapists, occupational therapists, social workers and dieticians
- carry out specialist procedures such as intra-articular joint injections
- undertake research
- educate other healthcare professionals.

SCHOOL NURSING

School nurses undertake health interviews, administer immunisation programmes, carry out developmental screening and provide health and sex education within the school. School nurses are employed either by a Primary Care Trust, NHS Trust in Wales, health board in Scotland, Health and Social Services Board in Northern Ireland or directly by the school, if it is independent.

SEXUAL HEALTH NURSING

Sexual health includes HIV, family planning and sexually transmitted disease services. Some clinics specialise in support and advice to young people under 26, including under-16s. Nurses working in sexual health:

- carry out health assessments
- undertake diagnostic tests
- provide pre- and post-test counselling
- provide information and advice about treatment
- educate clients through health promotion initiatives
- undertake outreach work in schools, colleges, youth projects and hostels, where relevant.

TELEPHONE ADVICE AND CONSULTATION

There are growing numbers of opportunities for nurses to provide information, advice and guidance over the telephone. NHS Direct is the largest telephone health advice and consultation service in the world and operates in England and Wales. Scotland has set up NHS 24.

NHS Direct

Nurses working for NHS Direct answer calls from the public and give advice on a wide range of health-related issues. They use a system of computer-based decision support guidelines to offer the appropriate advice, which can range from self-care to an emergency service referral.

NHS Direct sites also employ health information advisors, who give information about local health and social services, self-help groups, charities and common health conditions. All nurses recruited to NHS Direct in England will need to have attained the appropriate competencies, and the recruitment of disabled nurses or those who have retired due to ill health is encouraged.

Four or five years' post-registration experience is usually needed to become an NHS Direct Nurse Advisor. Many NHS Direct advisors have experience or hold a qualification in A&E nursing, but a full range of nursing expertise is represented in the NHS Direct workforce. Experience of assessing patients with undiagnosed and undifferentiated problems is useful.

Basic computer skills and knowledge of Windows-based products is useful but not essential as in-house training is provided. The initial NHS Direct training programme ranges from five to twelve weeks and covers telephone communication, call centre technology, the use of clinical protocols, clinical assessment, ethical issues and accountability.

Nurse advisors help callers to access appropriate healthcare or to manage their symptoms at home, by using computerised protocols. The role includes the opportunity to work on special projects, update information resources, develop policies and procedures and to liaise with key organisations. Experienced advisors act as preceptors and mentors to nurses new to the service.

There are opportunities to be seconded to the National Training Team and to deliver presentations and lectures to outside organisations. Career progression to a management, training or lead nurse position is possible, with some centres employing a consultant nurse.

In the voluntary sector many helplines are staffed by volunteers, but a number of major national helplines also employ nurses to provide specialist information and advice. They cover topics such as cancer, epilepsy, diabetes, asthma and support for older people. Such roles include writing relevant information materials and policy documents. The Medical Advisory Service (MAS) is a registered charity that employs nurses to provide professional advice and information over the telephone on all aspects of medical and healthcare matters. MAS have provided telephone helpline services for, among others, The Foundation for the Study of Infant Death, The Meningitis Research Foundation and the Irritable Bowel Syndrome Network. Several private healthcare companies provide helplines for subscribers to personal medical insurance. Nurses provide an information and advice service similar to that offered by NHS Direct and NHS 24.

THEATRE NURSING (PERIOPERATIVE NURSING)

Theatre nurses are responsible for the care and safety of patients undergoing surgical procedures. They play a central role in the pre-, intra- and post-operative phases of the patient's surgical experience. They ensure that the patient's rights and dignity are maintained throughout.

There are various specialist roles within the perioperative field:

- The anaesthetic nurse's role involves caring for the patient before, during and after the induction of anaesthesia. The anaesthetic nurse plays an important role in ensuring that the patient is having the correct procedure, that all relevant information is available and in reassuring the patient on their arrival in theatre. He or she also ensures that relevant equipment and medication is prepared and ready for use.

- The scrub nurse assists the surgeon(s) during the surgical procedure by preparing instruments and assisting in their use. Scrub nurses anticipate the requirements of the surgeon, pass correct instruments and ensure that nothing is left inside the patient during or after the operation. The circulating nurse is responsible for the environment outside the sterile field and assists in creating and maintaining a safe surgical environment.

- The recovery room nurse assesses, cares for and monitors the patient recovering from the immediate effects of surgery and anaesthesia. This includes monitoring vital signs, urine output, wound dressings and maintaining intravenous fluids. Interpersonal skills are used to reassure the patient as they awake from surgery. Assessment of pain and administration of relevant medication, through liaison with the anaesthetist, is also important. Communication of correct information to the ward or critical care staff is also essential to ensure appropriate continuing care of the patient when they leave the theatre environment. The first assistant in this role uses their specialist knowledge and skills to become more involved in risk management, infection control, wound management and suturing of wounds.

TROPICAL DISEASES

For queries relating to further training in the field of tropical disease, please contact: Hospital for Tropical Diseases, 4 St Pancras Way, London NW1 0PE. Tel: 020 7387 4411. Or: Liverpool School of Tropical Medicine, Pembroke Place, Liverpool L3 5QA. Tel: 0151 708 9393.

Such an enormous range of nursing opportunities! I used to think of a nurse as someone who worked on a ward with either adults or children – now I know better. What a choice. Or then again you might fancy the option of midwifery, where you can meet someone new every day. Want to know more?

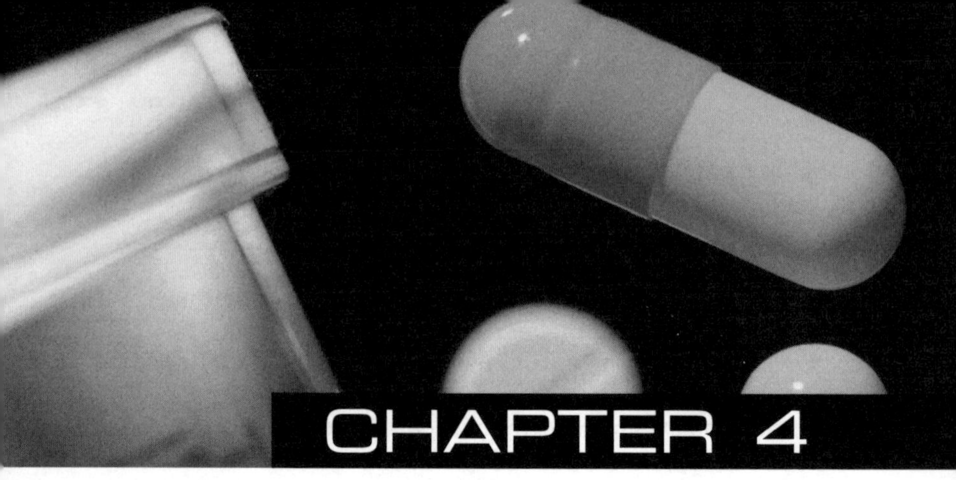

Where midwifery could take you

Being a midwife is about more than just delivering babies. It is about being with, supporting and caring for women, their partners and families from the early stages of pregnancy, through labour and delivery and into the first phase of postnatal care. Midwives are highly trained, multiskilled healthcare professionals. Though they work as part of a multidisciplinary team, liaising with other healthcare professionals, they enjoy a high level of responsibility and independence. Unless serious complications arise, a woman can expect to have all her antenatal (before the baby is born) and postnatal (after the baby is born) care needs met by midwives.

The role of the midwife is diverse. She:

- supports the mother and her family throughout the childbearing process to help them adjust to their parental role
- carries out clinical examinations
- provides health and parent education

- works in partnership with other health and social care services to meet the needs of individual mothers, such as teenage mothers, mothers who are socially excluded, disabled mothers and mothers from diverse ethnic backgrounds.

Because the midwife is present at every birth, whether at home or in hospital, she touches everyone's life. She is usually the first and main contact for the expectant mother during her pregnancy, and throughout labour and the post-natal period. She helps mothers to make informed choices about the services and options available to them by providing as much information as possible.

Midwives are responsible for their own individual practice and have a statutory responsibility to keep up to date with current knowledge. All midwives have a named Supervisor of Midwives to assist them with updating their knowledge and to ensure their practice is safe. It is the only profession that has supervision to protect the public from incompetent practitioners.

'I first trained as a nurse in Lincolnshire and then as a midwife in Suffolk. I have been a practising midwife since returning to work, after taking time off to have children, in 1987. During that time I have worked both in hospital and in the community and studied for a BSc degree in Midwifery. I was senior midwife in an integrated GP unit and very involved in the introduction of midwife-led care after the government's 'Changing Childbirth' report in 1993. My specialist area of midwifery is normality and low-risk care, and recently I've become increasingly interested in postnatal care.

'I love teaching parent education classes and since 1998 have been a midwife tutor, teaching Midwifery and Nursing Diploma and Degree students. Some of my time is spent as a clinical link lecturer and this is when I get to be with women. I have recently completed my training as a Supervisor of Midwives. I am passionate about midwifery and the place it has in this country in being "with women" throughout the special process of childbearing.'

Sally

Midwives work in all healthcare settings:

- in the maternity unit of a large general hospital
- in smaller stand-alone maternity units
- in private maternity hospitals
- in group practice
- at birth centres
- with general practitioners and in the community.

The majority of midwives work within the NHS, though it is possible to work privately and independently.

Midwives need to have a number of qualities in order to fulfil their role; the public expect a midwife to be:

- intuitive, kind, caring and objective
- able to act as an advocate for women and take responsibility for her own actions
- a good team player and work in partnership with other professionals
- flexible and adaptable to mothers' circumstances and needs
- prepared to look after all women, irrespective of class, creed, economic status, race or age
- professional and maintain accurate and contemporaneous records
- able to accept women and the circumstances in which they live.

CASE STUDY

Sherry Behan qualified in 1997 as a midwife after spending 20 years in teaching. 'My own experience of pregnancy and labour

prompted my change of career,' says Sherry. 'I had a bad first labour and birth and was left traumatised at the end. I didn't ever want any more children. But when I became pregnant the second time, the midwife made everything so much easier, I saw another side to the whole experience.' Following the birth of her second child, Sherry wanted to help improve the pregnancy and birth experience for other women. As she so quaintly says 'No one has to squat on a bucket and look at a pot plant any more. You can have what you like to make your pregnancy and labour easier.'

After a 20-year career as a teacher, Sherry retrained in 1994 and took a three-year Pre-Registration Diploma at the University of Brighton. She worked three days on a clinical ward and one day at college. 'The course was excellent – a balance of practical and academic work. I started with 3 weeks at college then 12 weeks in the community followed by time on the labour ward. I had to do 40 deliveries in order to qualify.' After qualifying, Sherry joined a midwifery bank to gain a spectrum of experience. Her first year was spent on the labour ward where she moved on to become a full-time E Grade midwife, then an F Grade Senior Staff midwife. 'I could go on to become a G Grade Senior midwife but that is more about ward management which isn't necessarily where I want to go. I would like to precept [teach] midwifery.'

When asked the recommended qualities of a midwife, Sherry highlighted stamina and a sense of humour. 'I took this job because I like to be with women. Pregnancy and labour are normal life events. It is my privileged role to help women deliver their baby safely and to walk out with a healthy baby. I see myself as an advocate for women, helping them to get what they need for the best birth possible.'

Midwives can develop their career in a variety of ways: taking on increased responsibility as a supervisor or manager of a ward or unit, becoming a clinical specialist, a consultant midwife, or perhaps moving into research or education. There are also many opportunities to work abroad. As your experience grows, you can research and develop special areas of practice and become involved in services such as family planning. There are opportunities to specialise in public health, women's health and to run specialist services, such as teenage pregnancy clinics.

'I qualified as a nurse in 1979 and a midwife in 1981. Over the next few years I gained experience as a midwife in both urban and rural settings. I became involved in research in 1987 while working as a midwife at Glasgow Royal Maternity Hospital. Since then I have been a midwife researcher involved in numerous studies into maternity care. My particular research interests have included hypertension in pregnancy, women's postnatal health and models of midwifery care.

'In 1992 I joined the research team at the Midwifery Development Unit (MDU) within Glasgow Royal Maternity Hospital. Following completion of the MDU study of midwife-managed care I remained within the unit as Practice Development Midwife. In July 2000 I joined NRIS for a nine-month secondment as clinical research fellow and in July 2001 I returned as a full-time member of the research team as research fellow on the Practitioner Decision Making programme.'

Helen

Midwifery is about caring for women and their families through an exciting and major life event. The midwife is often the key health professional supporting, guiding and caring for the woman and her growing baby through the nine months of pregnancy, during the birth itself and afterwards in the postnatal period.

Midwives provide woman-centred integrated care, which requires them to work shifts, day and night duty, be prepared to take on-call rotas and travel between hospital or institution and mother's home. From April 2002, newly qualified NHS midwives' starting salary is £17,000, and £31,000 can be earned after five years' experience.

Midwifery is a challenging career and its duties wide-ranging: from carrying out clinical examinations, providing advice on diet, parenting, infant feeding, etc., providing emotional support, running antenatal classes, assisting births and administering pain-relief drugs to the monitoring of both healthy and special-care newborns.

Midwives work shift patterns to provide continual support for women day and night. Midwives do not make decisions for women but are there to provide the right support and information so that women can make their own informed choices about the care they receive before, during and after pregnancy and labour.

Midwives also work with other healthcare professionals on initiatives such as improving breastfeeding rates and promoting health during pregnancy and afterwards.

Every delivery is a major event in the lives of the people involved. Midwives have the lead professional role in preparing for and managing the event, intervening where necessary and knowing what to do if the mother or baby is sick. Having babies happens to all sorts of people, so you will be providing professional support and reassurance to a huge diversity of women, during one of the most emotionally intense periods in their lives. You will have to stay calm and alert in times of stress, and enable women to feel confident and in control. On the rare occasions when something goes wrong, you have to be ready to react quickly and effectively.

Midwives offer individual care to women and their families and help them take part in their own care planning during pregnancy. Both during and after pregnancy you will be with the woman in her own locality. Midwifery is as much about supporting the woman and her partner, as helping with the birth of the baby. Support continues from the confirmation of the pregnancy up to 28 days after the baby's birth.

COMMUNITY MIDWIFERY

Community midwives first see women after about ten weeks of pregnancy and continue to provide care either in the doctor's surgery or at the woman's home. During the antenatal period (before the baby is born) midwives offer: screening, full antenatal surveillance, parent education, advice on all issues relating to pregnancy, information on choices for labour and delivery and discussion regarding infant feeding. After the birth, community midwives provide care and support in the parents' home.

INDEPENDENT MIDWIFERY

Independent midwives (IMs) are fully qualified midwives who have chosen to work outside the NHS in a self-employed capacity. The role encompasses the care of women during pregnancy, birth and afterwards.

Midwifery is the most securely regulated profession in the UK. All practising midwives must adhere to the Midwives Rules, as set out in the 1902 Midwives Act of Parliament and subsequent amendments. All independent midwives are subject to yearly supervisory visits and equipment checks and must notify their NHS appointed Supervisor of Midwives of their 'Intention to Practise' each April. In line with the requirements of their regulatory body, the Nursing and Midwifery Council (NMC, see page 105 for details), IMs are required to ensure that their clinical practice is up to date and that their actions are within their sphere of competence.

'I have been in midwifery since 1974 and have worked in the NHS, the Middle East and midwifery education. I was a midwife in the army before working in the NHS. The numbers of women who had induced labours in the NHS, and the assumption that women would have an epidural, surprised me. High levels of induction of labour and the way women were expected to have epidurals came as a shock and so after a while I went to work in Israel and later I also worked in the United Arab Emirates, running a newly opened maternity unit.

'When I returned to England I worked as a midwifery sister and also as a midwifery lecturer. I felt midwifery education was taking me further away from practice, so I returned to the NHS until becoming an independent midwife in 1996. I thoroughly enjoy working as an independent midwife and like having time to spend with women, instead of feeling rushed. I also like being able to get to know women and their partners and having time to involve them in the care. I'm still doing some teaching – at South Bank University – alongside my independent practice.'

Sharon, independent midwife

IMs offer continuity of care, and empower women to make informed choices and decisions at every stage. IM bookings are often for home births, and the rest are for planned hospital births. IMs liaise with other healthcare practitioners if and when necessary. They can arrange all screenings and diagnostic tests, such as scans and blood tests, either through the NHS or privately. Should the desired place of birth or type of care need to change at any time, IMs can assist clients in achieving this as smoothly and gently as possible. IMs accompany their clients into all hospitals, their roles depending on local arrangements and clients' needs.

Midwives have a client group who are on the whole very healthy, and in need of help and advice only because they are expecting a baby. The birth itself may be at the heart of the process, but midwives provide support to women, their babies, their partners and families, from conception to the first phase of postnatal care.

CASE STUDY

Andrya Prescott, Surrey Independent Midwives
'I am part of a team providing comprehensive midwifery care to the women in Surrey and Hampshire and also into South London and West Sussex. I am registered to practise with the NMC, and abide by the Midwives Rules and Code of Practice. I am also a member of the Royal College of Midwives (RCM), the Independent Midwives Association (IMA), the Association of Radical Midwives (ARM) and the Association for Improvements in Maternity Services (AIMS).

'I have been an independent midwife since January 1999 attending women for their home births, water births, twin births, breech births, home births after caesarean (HBAC), healing births after previous traumatic experiences, first babies, ninth babies, and those in between, in Hampshire, Surrey, West Sussex and southwest London.

'I am passionate about midwifery and love working with women and families, whether their situation is challenging or straightforward. My dedication to midwifery would not be possible without the support and love of my husband Steve. We live in Godalming with our cats.

'I became a midwife after a good friend had said she was thinking of either becoming a healthcare worker or a midwife. That was it for me – I knew it was my calling. To work with women and their families at such an amazing time, to help them have the experience they wanted . . . However, I was 19 at the time and felt that I needed to spend a bit more time thinking about midwifery and what it would mean to me and so waited a few years before I finally applied. In the meantime I worked in bookshops, feeding my book addiction!

'Once I applied and was accepted at King's College London to my three-year direct entry midwifery course, my life turned round dramatically. I had truly found my vocation. I passed with a distinction and so, with plenty of encouragement and support for my plans to become independent, I moved down to Hampshire and set up my practice as an independent midwife. After a year or so of working alone, I began to provide back-up work to Andrea Dombrowe and Jane Westbrook and they then invited me to join them as Surrey Independent Midwives. It was a wonderful opportunity for mutual support and skill sharing as well as providing our clients with a collection of midwives that could be called on at any time, allowing each of us to take holiday from our pagers every now and again.

'So here I am, enjoying the variety that each family I work with brings, lecturing about my passion occasionally and helping women to birth safely and to know that they did all they could for themselves and their baby.'

WHAT ARE THE FUTURE PROSPECTS?

Midwives have an opportunity to work in different healthcare settings, and gain experience in all aspects of caring for mothers and babies. They have an option to develop their midwifery career in many different ways. It may be as a clinical specialist – a consultant midwife, or in management as a head of midwifery services or supervisor of midwives at local authority level. Some midwives prefer to pursue an academic career in education and research. Midwives have developed innovative specialist roles, in ultrasound, foetal medicine, intensive care neonatal units, public health, parenting education and many others. The opportunities are endless in the health service. There are also opportunities for midwives to work in the European Community or with Voluntary Service Overseas.

Great stuff. You could go into nursing. You could go into midwifery. So what about the training? How does that work? Move on.

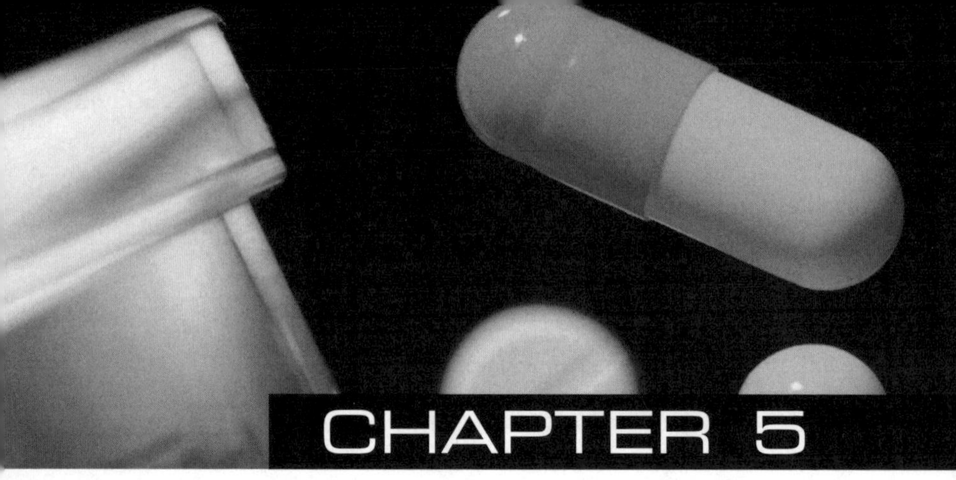

Getting into nursing and midwifery

THE TWO ROUTES TO QUALIFICATION

PRE-REGISTRATION (FOR NEW STARTERS)

To qualify as a nurse in the UK, you have to be accepted for entry onto the Professional Register. Either the degree or the diploma route will take you there.

1. Diploma of Higher Education in Nursing (DipHE Nursing)

   These programmes integrate equal amounts of theoretical study and supervised nursing practice. On completion, students are awarded both an academic and a professional qualification. Supervised nursing practice takes place in both hospital and community settings. Programmes normally last three years: a 12-month Common Foundation Programme (CFP) followed by around two years in one of the four branches of nursing – Adult, Mental Health, Learning Disabilities or Children's Nursing. Minimum entry is five GCSEs or equivalent.

2 Pre-Registration Nursing degree

As above. Some degree programmes last for four years. Minimum entry is five GCSEs, plus two A-levels.

3 Accelerated Diploma programmes (for graduates with a health-related degree)

These shortened programmes, comprising 50 per cent theory and 50 per cent practice, are modified from existing DipHE Nursing programmes and lead to qualification in Adult, Mental Health, Learning Disabilities or Children's Nursing. Accelerated programmes last at least 24 months: at least six months in the CFP and at least 18 months in the appropriate branch programme.

On completion of any of the above courses, you register your qualification with the NMC, enabling you to practise.

Note: Applicants will need to complete the degree programme should they wish to apply for senior level positions or work in education or management in the future.

POST-REGISTRATION

Post-registration provides a learning route for qualified practitioners who wish to accumulate credit to gain a degree.

HEALTH

You have to complete a health questionnaire when you apply for nurse or midwifery training and will be asked to identify any special needs related to a disability. Your acceptance on a course will be subject to satisfactory health clearance. If you have a disability, you may find it useful to contact Skill (The National Bureau for Students with Disabilities), on 0800 328 5050, or visit their website at www.skill.org.uk.

NURSING

Sweeping changes have been made to student nurse training since Project 2000 was introduced in the early 1990s. Previously, nursing and midwifery training had been carried out within a school of nursing at a hospital site where the nurses both studied and worked on the wards. Qualified nurses became state registered nurses or registered general nurses (RGNs) and were registered with the NMC. A second, shorter and more practical, training concluded with qualification as an enrolled nurse.

The aim of Project 2000 was to professionalise nursing by transferring nurse training into higher education, within a university setting. Nurses were encouraged to study to diploma or degree level, enrolled nurse training stopped and schools of nursing could no longer be found within a hospital. Hospitals had to pay universities for the education and training of student nurses, and in turn the universities would provide nurses who were academically sound and fit for practice.

Until Project 2000, many of the ward workforce were first-, second- and third-year student nurses, who were on the ward rota and part of the ward team. With the introduction of Project 2000, student nurses became just that – students. They spent most of their time studying and less time on ward work gaining practical experience. To fill the resulting gap in the workforce the government increased the number of healthcare assistants (non- or semi-trained care staff).

NURSING COURSES WITH SOMETHING DIFFERENT

European Nursing

University of Brighton	01273 600900
Middlesex University	020 8411 5898

Nursing & Social Work Studies (Learn Disab) with RN/DipSW

Nursing Science

University of Hertfordshire	01707 284800
University of Nottingham	0115 951 5151

Almost every university runs a programme of study for nurse training, usually within its department of health or life sciences. Both the diploma and the degree level courses now take three academic years. The entry requirements for the diploma and the degree course differ and prospective students should contact the university of their choice for details.

DIPLOMA OR DEGREE?
Diploma and degree courses in nursing are run at different academic levels, but there is some overlap. Diploma level students can transfer to degree courses or can opt to come back and top up their diploma in nursing to a degree at a later stage. Whether you do a diploma or a degree in nursing depends largely on your qualifications on entry. Whichever course you decide to take, you will begin work as a D grade staff nurse on the same salary.

ENTRY REQUIREMENTS

The minimum entry requirements are given below, but many universities will require you to hold more than the minimum, including A-levels:

- five GCSEs/GCE O-levels, grade C or above (including English and a science/maths subject for entry to midwifery); or
- five CSEs grade 1; or
- five SCEs grade 1 (Scotland); or
- five SCE ordinary, grades A–C (Scotland); or
- GNVQ Intermediate level plus one GCSE/GCE O-level, grade A–C; or
- GNVQ Advanced Level or NVQ level 3; or
- SVQ level 3; GSVQ level 3 (Scotland); or
- SVQ level 2 (Scotland) if the programme began after September 2000
- a Kitemarked Access to Higher Education course; or
- Edexcel Foundation (BTEC) National or Higher National Diploma; or

- passes in the Northern Ireland Grammar School Senior Certificate of Education;
- a qualification awarded by the Nursery Nursing Education Board (NNEB) dating from 1985, including the Diploma in Post-Qualifying Studies.

If you don't have the minimum entry requirement, your training options are:

- *Access to Higher Education courses (one to two years)*

  These are designed to enable students aged 21 and over from under-represented groups to enter higher education. People without formal prior qualifications, or who wish to return to study after a break, are particularly encouraged to apply. As well as the generic programmes, there are also programmes that are designed to lead to a specific named route within higher education, e.g. Access to Nursing. Programmes are normally taken over one year full time, or two years part time. Most of the programmes are run by further education colleges, but your local adult education centre, community centre or university may also provide them.

- *The UKCC DC Test*

  These tests are designed to enable people who do not otherwise satisfy the minimum statutory entry requirements to undertake pre-registration nursing or midwifery programmes. The tests cover areas such as numerical ability, verbal/non-verbal reasoning and English comprehension. An information booklet (cost £2.00) is available from institutions offering the tests or from: Nurse Selection Project, School of Education, University of Leeds, Leeds LS2 9JT. Tel: 01132 334672.

- *Nurse Cadet Scheme (two years)*

  This scheme was introduced to strengthen and widen access to pre-registration nursing and midwifery education. It enables people without prior formal qualifications to train within the hospital setting to a standard considered appropriate for entry into a pre-registration course. Run by various NHS trusts in England, this scheme enables you to undertake an initial training programme, successful completion of which gives you an NVQ level 3 or Access to Nursing qualification. You are then seconded to a nearby university to take a nursing diploma course, leading to registration as a nurse.

If you have at least five GCSEs at grade C or above (including English language) you must first undertake a Pre-Registration Nursing Diploma course. You should check with the individual institution for their specific entry requirements, but in all cases you will be required to be at least 17 years old when the course starts. For all Pre-Registration Diplomas in Nursing you should apply through the Nursing and Midwifery Admissions Services (NMAS) (see page 106 for contact details).

Although nursing courses increasingly prefer candidates with a science background, most nursing students still do not have the types or levels of qualifications required to do medicine. The current minimum entry requirements for a nursing diploma are five GCSEs at grade C or above (or equivalent), although most entrants have higher qualifications, such as degrees. Therefore, nurses who want to study medicine usually need further qualifications to fulfil the entry criteria. The options are either studying for appropriate A-levels or looking at alternatives such as a premedical course. For this you need to have good A-level grades, although these need not be science-related. A degree in nursing can be used for entry into medicine, although most medical schools will require additional science-based academic qualifications, such as A-levels in chemistry and biology.

The one-year premedical course is currently offered by eight medical schools (Bristol, Dundee, Edinburgh, Manchester, Newcastle, Wales College of Medicine, Sheffield and King's College London). Successful completion of the course automatically gives you entry into first-year medicine. The courses vary widely, from those designed specifically for medicine, and therefore with an emphasis on the biological sciences, to those that allocate students to foundation science courses already in place.

COURSES IN EXPEDITION MEDICINE

Expedition Medicine Ltd provide a variety of courses aimed at enabling medics to develop the essential skills which will allow them to feel confident practising medicine alone and in hostile environments. They provide three courses run both in the UK and abroad and developed for medics at different stages of their training.

Their two-day course was developed in conjunction with Raleigh International and was aimed at House Officers and nurses who need to develop the practical skills essential for expedition medicine. The four-day course, which is more comprehensive, assumes a certain level of ability and experience and is aimed at doctors and nurses with A&E experience. In addition to UK courses, Expedition Medicine run a very exciting course in the Arctic, aimed at preparing medics for working as an expedition medic in cold hostile environments and at altitude. For further information contact Expedition Medicine Ltd on 01460 30456, or look at the website: www.expeditionmedicine.co.uk.

In order to train as a health visitor, you must first qualify as a nurse and have gained ideally at least two years' practice. An employer seconds most health visitor students onto a programme, although a few people may fund themselves. In addition, information about funding and general information may be obtained from the Community Practitioners and Health Visitors Association (CPHVA) and the local Workforce Development Confederation (WDC). Further information: Community Practitioners and Health Visitors Association, 40 Bermondsey Street, London SE1 3UD. Tel: 020 7939 7000. Website: www.amicus-cphva.org.

NURSE TRAINING

- Currently, training to be a nurse is a three-year degree or diploma course. Some schools of nursing offer two-year, 'fast track' courses for graduates with science degrees

- At the end of the course, you start work at the level of a D grade staff nurse
- The career ladder then progresses through the alphabet, with an E grade being a senior staff nurse, F grade being a junior sister, and so on, until H and I grades, which include nurse specialist and senior management positions
- In a similar way to doctors, nurses in more junior positions can switch around and work in different areas, specialising later on in their career.

MIDWIFERY

If you know from the outset that you want to be a midwife, you can take a direct entry diploma or degree programme lasting three or four years. Alternatively, you can qualify as a registered nurse (RN) then undertake a 78-week programme into midwifery.

All programmes are 50 per cent theory, taught in universities (see www.nmas.ac.uk for institutions offering diploma courses in midwifery studies and www.ucas.com for universities offering the degree course) and 50 per cent clinical practice in local hospitals (and the community) linked with the university. Universities offering midwifery education are also listed on NHS careers website (www.nhs.uk/careers).

'I love every minute of my (midwifery) course and have just completed a three-week placement within the hospital. I had plenty of experiences and the midwives I worked with were great. The greatest experience of all was my very first delivery. This was something that I have been desperate to do since starting the course. I did wonder whether I would feel afraid or nervous when the time actually came, but I didn't. I felt really confident and totally at ease with the situation. I love being with the women during their labours and feel totally overjoyed when they experience the birth they desire.'

Amanda

Successful completion of either programme means you are a qualified midwife and you will be officially registered with the NMC. In addition, you qualify with a degree or diploma. Diploma programmes require 60 credits of study at level 3, whereas the degree programme requires 120 credits. This means the degree course is more intense, including additional modules in research and a dissertation. In choosing between the two programmes, candidates should consider their desired qualification outcome and their own academic strength. A diploma can be topped-up to a degree at a later date with further study. For some institutions all candidates enter at diploma level and choose to switch to the degree after the first or possibly second year.

As far as programme content goes, there is little variation between institutions as professional registration has standard study requirements. Wherever you study you can expect to follow modules in anatomy and physiology, behavioural science, clinical midwifery skills, nutrition, infant feeding and handling complexities in childbirth, as well as touching on sociology, psychology, law, ethics, research skills and more besides. However, institutions may vary in their methods of teaching and assessment. For clinical practice, some programmes require you to experience working in two or three different hospitals, while others send you to just one for the duration of the course. View the universities' own websites for specific programme information.

'I am a third-year student midwife on clinical placement at a midwifery-led unit, and over the last two days I have been lucky enough to care for two labouring women. The first was a mother who had had a previous long, augmented labour and delivery with an epidural. She arrived on the unit contracting well, entered the birthing pool at 8cm dilated and progressed to a normal water-birth delivery, which she was extremely happy to experience. The second birth was a home birth. She laboured well and gave birth to a 4,550g baby with ease and no stitches. I had had a lot of contact with this woman, so being present at the birth was a very fulfilling moment for me and it really gave me a boost (I know I am making the right career move).

'I work in a midwifery-led unit which offers antenatal, intrapartum and postnatal care to women, with a birthing

pool available, and it supports a large percentage of home deliveries. The unit is a part of a larger consultant-led unit 20 miles away and is supported by a local GP practice. As a student I have spent the first 18 months of my course based here and it has been an invaluable part of my development as it has shown me normal midwifery right from the start. I have now returned as a senior student and love it and would ideally like to practise here once qualified.'

Louise

ENTRY REQUIREMENTS

DIPLOMA LEVEL

Five GCSEs at grades A–C (including English and Maths and one science subject). Alternative qualifications are:

- Double Award Vocational A-level
- NVQ level 3
- BTEC National
- Access to Higher Education course

Admission to diploma courses in England is made through the NMAS, and students are paid a non-means-tested bursary during their course. You receive a Diploma and a Registered Midwife qualification.

DEGREE ROUTE

The minimum requirement for degree courses is two A-levels. Science is one of the preferred subjects. Application to the degree route is through UCAS. You will gain a degree and Registered Midwife qualification.

Entry is very competitive, and many students have higher than minimum requirements. Each university has its own criteria, so it is best to check with the individual institution.

ABOUT THE COURSE AND QUALIFICATIONS

Both diploma and degree courses are organised to give you both the theoretical background and hands-on practical experience with women and their families. The course lasts three to four years. You can access shortened midwifery courses following a nursing qualification if you prefer to do a nursing course first.

The midwifery course is organised in modules, which include biological sciences, applied sociology and psychology, professional practice and others. Each module is assessed, usually through continuous assignments, but examinations may form part of assessments.

Practising midwives must be registered with the statutory body for nursing, midwifery and health visiting. This is the Nursing and Midwifery Council, NMC (see page 105 for details). The Council maintains a register of midwives. To remain on it, midwives must update their knowledge and maintain a professional portfolio as evidence of their updating. To enable the Council to know which midwives are practising, all practising midwives must notify their intention to practise on an annual basis.

INFORMATION

For course information on midwifery including Degree combined with Midwifery (three years), Degree combined with Midwifery (four years) and Diploma of Higher Education (DipHE) in Midwifery, visit NHS Careers at: www.nhscareers.nhs.uk/nhs-knowledge_base/data/1420.html

HOW APPLICATIONS THROUGH NMAS AND UCAS DIFFER

UCAS APPLICATIONS

UCAS is the central organisation that processes applications for full-time undergraduate courses at UK universities and colleges. See page 106 for more details.

NMAS APPLICATIONS

The Nursing and Midwifery Admissions Service (NMAS) is an agency which acts on behalf of the Department of Health to process applications for full-length, diploma-level, pre-registration nursing and midwifery programmes at universities and colleges of higher education in England. NMAS does not process applications for degrees in nursing or midwifery, shortened programmes for qualified nurses or midwives and post-registration programmes. Other applications not processed by NMAS are courses offered by institutions outside England and adaptation programmes for nurses or midwives who qualified outside the UK. For contact details, see page 106.

In choosing a university you need to think about the following questions:

- Do I want to stay at home to study or move away? Can I afford to move away? If so, where would I like to live? Big city? Small city? Region?
- What kind of university would I prefer? Campus? What is the reputation of the institution or faculty?
- What facilities do the various universities provide? Library resources? Sports facilities?
- How is the course organised and taught, e.g. problem-based learning?
- Which hospitals are the universities linked to? Can I choose where I want to go for my clinical placement? How many different locations will I practise in?
- If I start following the diploma course is it possible to switch to the degree or top up later?

Further information is available from the following organisations:

The NHS Student Grants Unit, Room 212c Government Buildings, Norcross, Blackpool FY5 3TA. Tel: 01253 655655 (diploma enquiries). Tel: 01253 333314 (degree enquiries).

Scotland
The Students Awards Agency for Scotland, 3 Redheughs Rigg, South Gyle, Edinburgh EH12 9HH. Tel: 0131 4768212.

Wales
NHS Wales Student Award Unit, 2nd Floor, Golate House, 101 St Mary Street, Cardiff CF10 1DX. Tel: 029 2026 1495.

Northern Ireland
The Department of Higher and Further Education Training and Employment, Student Support Branch, 4th Floor Adelaide House, 39–49 Adelaide Street, Belfast BT2 8FD. Tel: 028 9025 7777.

Or contact:
NHS Student Grants, Department of Health, PO Box 777, London SE1 6XH. Email: doh@prologistics.co.uk.
Website: www.doh.gov.uk/hcsmain.htm.

There is a central application process for both degree and diploma programmes.
For diploma programmes you will need to apply to:
The Nursing and Midwifery Admissions Service (NMAS).
See page 106 for details.
For degree programmes you will need to apply to:
The Universities and Colleges Admissions Service (UCAS).
See page 106 for details.

COURSES IN TROPICAL MEDICINE
A course in Tropical Medicine is often valuable for those wishing to work overseas, and may be a requirement for nursing in developing countries. The London School of Hygiene and Tropical Medicine offers the Diploma in Tropical Nursing, which runs twice a year from March to July and from September to February. The course is one day per week and lasts for 19 weeks. It is available to registered nurses only.

The content includes emergency midwifery, dentistry, water and sanitation technology and mental health in the developing world, together with wide coverage of clinical tropical medicine and primary healthcare. Practical skills and laboratory work are also included. Peter Wilson, London School of Hygiene and Tropical Medicine, Keppel Street, London WC1 7HT. Tel: 020 7927 2627. Website: www.lshtm.ac.uk.

For more information, see *The Directory of Nursing and Midwifery Courses* published by Trotman, www.trotman.co.uk.

So what's it to be – nursing or midwifery? Still not sure? Want to know how you can make these careers even more fascinating and really be at the cutting edge of healthcare? Let's go and see.

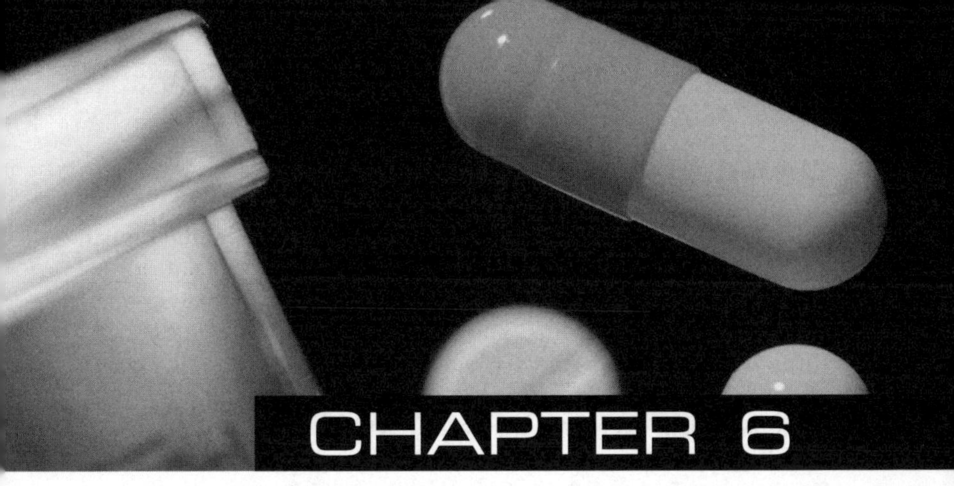

Complementary therapies in nursing and midwifery

Complementary medicine is a wide-ranging group of healthcare systems and practices that is not considered part of conventional Western medicine based on scientific knowledge of anatomy, phsyiology and chemical remedies.

Complementary therapies are used in conjunction with conventional medicine (e.g. aromatherapy to ease discomfort after surgery) and are based upon traditional knowledge contained within complete systems of theory and practice that have evolved over time.

Complementary therapies should not be seen as an alternative to orthodox medicine, but as a valuable support that recognises the emotional and spiritual as well as the physical aspects of healing.

CASE STUDY

Yola Wright wanted to get away from home after spending much of her teenage years looking after a parent with psychiatric problems. 'I was 15 at the time and one day I just woke up and knew nursing was for me,' she says. In those days, you needed three GCEs, and Yola had six, but she couldn't start training until she was 18. However, she was able to study human biology and hygiene, which exempted her from Part 1 of her nursing training. Yola then moved on to Pre-Nursing and then to Preliminary Training School for three years after which she was qualified as an SRN. She did much of her training at the Royal Sussex County Hospital.

As a follow-up, she did six months of midwifery training in Mayday Hospital, Croydon. She then worked at Hove General Hospital in the private ward dealing with patients suffering from burns, cancer and a wide range of other conditions and worked her way up to become a staff nurse. During this time Yola married and gave birth to a son who had severe learning difficulties. For the next 20 years, she gave up her career to care for her son, making continued use of her nursing skills. As the years passed, Yola did various jobs 'I went into tropical fish tank maintenance and at another point even became a painter's model to earn some money.' As her son became more independent, Yola was offered a position as a courier for the Family Practitioner Committee, which gave her insight into another area of healthcare.

From this, she decided to become a practice nurse. She took a training course specifically for practice nurses, which built on her SRN skills. 'Not many practice nurses are full time,' says Yola, 'but I had a fascinating and wide range of conditions to work with at the GP's surgery. I dealt with asthma, diabetes, smears, changing of dressings, clinical work, health education and immunisation.' Yola was then approaching retirement but still wanted to do some hands-on work. 'I used to massage my son so I thought I would take an ITEC (International Therapy Examination Council) Anatomy and Physiology course which also included massage. Then I went on to take an IFPA (International Federation of Professional Aromatherapists) course.'

Following these qualifications, Yola continued working at the GP's surgery as a practice nurse and set up her aromatherapy clinic there. When she retired, she was approached by the Nigel Porter Unit at the Royal Sussex County Hospital where they treat women with breast cancer, and was asked if she would provide an aromatherapy service to the women, which she was happy to do alongside her own private aromatherapy practice. Now 65, Yola is having some well-deserved time off. 'I would recommend any person wanting to come into nursing to concentrate first on getting their nursing degree. Then, when you are happy with the overall direction of your career, you can bolt-on a complementary therapy such as aromatherapy.'

When asked the qualities a practice nurse most needs, Yola said 'A sense of humour and an interest in people because you get to know whole families. I would add tolerance as well because people can do the oddest things. A calm attitude and good time management as well. Unflappability and patience are also important.'

ALTERNATIVE AND COMPLEMENTARY MEDICINES AND THERAPIES

Surveys over the past decade have reflected a growing public demand for, and interest by health practitioners (doctors and nurses) in, reliable, practical and safe natural medicines, especially where conventional treatments are ineffective. Alternative and complementary medicines and therapies are rapidly becoming integrated within GP practices, health centres and hospitals. In 1993 a survey conducted by the British Market Research Bureau found that 89 per cent of the population would use complementary medicine. GPs have also become more inclined to recommend non-conventional treatments. Last year, Baroness Cumberlege, the Department of Health minister responsible for complementary medicine, reported that 40 per cent of registered medical practitioners delegate patients to complementary medical treatments.

Other surveys have shown that medical students, doctors and nurses are now actively studying and using alternative and complementary medicines. Studies have indicated that as many as 70 per cent of hospital doctors and 93 per cent of GPs have referred patients to non-conventional health practitioners. Twenty per cent of GPs and 12 per cent of hospital doctors actually practise some form of complementary medicine, and 85 per cent of medical students, 76 per cent of GPs and 69 per cent of hospital doctors feel that complementary therapies should be made available on the NHS.

Homoeopathy is unique among all of the alternative and complementary therapies, as it has been part of the National Health Service since 1948 and is available at five NHS homoeopathic hospitals: The Royal London, Glasgow, Liverpool (Mossley Hill), Bristol and Tunbridge Wells. The Queen is patron of the Royal London Homoeopathic Hospital NHS Trust, and the royal family have employed homoeopathic physicians for generations. Other therapies can also be made available but largely at the discretion of District Health Authorities (DHAs) or Family Health Service Authorities (FHSAs). In 1992, a national survey carried out among DHAs, FHSAs and GP fundholding practices found that 70 per cent wanted complementary therapies (mostly homoeopathy, acupuncture, osteopathy and chiropractic) to be available on the NHS, and 83 per cent of DHAs, although most have incorporated them on an experimental basis.

Many FHSAs have regarded health promotion clinics as a means of employing complementary therapies for smoking cessation, stress management and pain. The main barriers to more widespread application of complementary therapies are lack of information about the therapies, lack of available evidence relating to their effectiveness and lack of resources.

COMPLEMENTARY THERAPIES IN THE NHS

- **75% of the public want alternative therapies made available on the NHS.**
- **45% of registered medical practitioners refer patients to complementary medical treatments.**
- **85% of medical students, 76% of GPs and 69% of hospital doctors feel that complementary therapies should be made available on the NHS.**

- 58% of nurses incorporate or use alternative therapies in their work, and 89% recommend alternative therapies to patients.

www.internethealthlibrary.com/Surveys/surveys-uk-comp-therapies-nhs.htm

The General Medical Council's position has long been clear: any family doctor may employ a complementary therapist to offer treatment on the NHS so long as the doctor retains clinical responsibility and accountability (Department of Health press release, 3 December 1991; *Hansard* 200, 3 December 1991).

More and more people are using complementary therapies – one in five of the population now, according to the BBC. With over 50,000 practitioners and a £1.6 billion per year valuation, complementary therapies are an important part of the health sector. However, most of this provision is outside the NHS, with well over 90 per cent of complementary therapies purchased privately.

NEW GUIDELINES ON COMPLEMENTARY THERAPIES

The National Council has published guidelines on the practice of complementary therapies for palliative care for Hospice and Specialist Palliative Care Services and The Prince of Wales's Foundation for Integrated Health. The publication aims to improve the quality of complementary therapies in palliative care and guarantee patient safety.

'These guidelines address issues which are directly related to patient safety in the provision of complementary therapy services, including clinical governance, regulation and training of therapists and audit and evaluation,' writes Professor Mike Richards, the Department of Health's National Cancer Director, in a preface to the guidelines.

Public health minister Hazel Blears launched the guidelines on 9 June 2003, announcing that free copies would be given to all UK hospices, supportive and palliative care providers and primary care trusts.

> Guidance is offered on a number of therapies including acupuncture, aromatherapy, homeopathy, hypnosis and hypnotherapy, massage, reflexology, reiki, spiritual healing and therapeutic touch. Although the main focus is on cancer, the guidelines also look at how therapies can help with motor neurone disease, Parkinson's disease and multiple sclerosis.
>
> The guidelines aim to encourage managers, health professionals and others involved in developing complementary therapy services in palliative care to develop their own policies based on good practice and local needs.
>
> Around a third of cancer patients receive complementary therapy treatments, and almost half of those who do not receive them would like to do so. Complementary therapies can help cancer patients control stress, pain and the side effects of treatment. According to Professor Richards, many cancer patients choose to receive complementary therapies alongside conventional cancer treatments.
>
> Nursing and Midwifery Council, June 2003

In parts of the NHS there is combined provision of conventional and complementary services, e.g. in cancer services at Hammersmith Hospitals Trust or the Glastonbury Health Centre complementary medicine service.

FASCINATING FACT

The most commonly used therapies available within the NHS are acupuncture, aromatherapy, chiropractic, homoeopathy, hypnotherapy and osteopathy.

AUTHOR'S NOTE: I'm a qualified reflexologist, nutritionist and stress management therapist and work with breast cancer patients in my clinic with patients referred to me by the NHS. Shortly I'll be working within an NHS breast care unit one afternoon a week delivering relaxation therapies to women waiting for breast surgery. Integrated healthcare services do happen! I also know of an NHS healthcare worker working full time within a major cancer centre running two clinics a week in massage and aromatherapy, and a nurse with a community health background currently working as a discharge planning nurse and working part time doing Indian head massage in a breast care unit. More integrated healthcare is happening within a district nursing team where one nurse has recently qualified as an aromatherapist and another is learning reiki.

COMPLEMENTARY THERAPY OVERVIEW

Acupuncture	Acupuncture is a treatment involving fine needles, which can relieve symptoms of some physical and psychological conditions and may encourage the patient's body to heal and repair itself. Acupuncture stimulates the nerves in skin and muscle and can produce a variety of effects. It increases the body's release of natural painkillers – endorphin and serotonin – in the pain pathways of both the spinal cord and the brain, which modifies the way pain signals are received. Modern research shows that acupuncture can affect most of the body's systems – the nervous system, muscle tone, hormone outputs, circulation, antibody production and allergic responses, as well as the respiratory, digestive, urinary and reproductive systems.
Aromatherapy	This can be defined as the art and science of utilising naturally extracted aromatic essences from plants to balance, harmonise and promote the health of body, mind and spirit – most commonly used in massage.
Chiropractic	Chiropractors treat problems with your joints, bones and muscles, and the effects they have on your nervous system. Working on all the

	joints of your body, particularly the spine, they use their hands to make often gentle, specific adjustments (the chiropractic word for manipulation) to improve the efficiency of your nervous system and release your body's natural healing ability.
Homoeopathy	Homoeopathy is an effective and scientific system of healing, using remedies, which assists the natural tendency of the body to heal itself. It recognises that all symptoms of ill health are expressions of disharmony within the whole person and that it is the patient, not the disease, that needs treatment.

ALTERNATIVE THERAPIES BACKED BY NICE
A government watchdog has backed the use of some complementary therapies in the treatment of multiple sclerosis (MS). Guidance from the National Institute for Clinical Excellence (NICE) says that doctors should let patients know about the possible benefits of t'ai chi, magnetic field therapy, massage and reflexology.

Complementary treatments are widely used by MS patients seeking relief from pain, fatigue and other symptoms. The guidance says that doctors should tell sufferers that there is 'some evidence to suggest' that the specified treatments might have benefits, even if there is not enough evidence to make firm recommendations.

However, many other popular treatments, including acupuncture, yoga, herbal remedies and aromatherapy, have failed to win NICE recognition. NICE also says that, whatever therapy patients choose to pursue, they should be encouraged to tell doctors about it.

It is understood that another clinical guideline expected soon – for treating depression – will also acknowledge a place for complementary therapy.

The NMC's Code of Professional Conduct states: 'You must ensure that the use of complementary or alternative therapies is safe and in the interests of patients and clients. This must be discussed with the team as part of the therapeutic process and the patient or client must consent to their use.' For more detailed guidance, see the Advice section of the website (under 'Complementary and alternative therapies').

Nursing and Midwifery Council, November 2003

Hypnotherapy

Psychological therapy and counselling is the treatment of emotional and psychological disorders, unwanted habits and undesirable feelings, using psychological techniques alone. The aim of all such therapy is to help people find meaningful alternatives to their present unsatisfactory ways of thinking, feeling or behaving. Therapy also tends to help clients become more accepting both of themselves and of others and can be most useful in promoting personal development and unlocking inner potential.

There are many forms of psychological therapy; hypnotherapy is distinctive in that it attempts to address the client's subconscious mind. In practice, the hypnotherapist often requires the client to be in a relaxed state, frequently enlists the power of the client's own imagination and may utilise a wide range of techniques from story telling, metaphor or symbolism to the use of direct suggestions for beneficial change.

Analytical techniques may also be employed in an attempt to uncover problems deemed to lie in a client's past, or therapy may concentrate more on a client's current life and presenting problems. It is generally considered helpful if

	the client is personally motivated to change (rather than relying solely on the therapist's efforts) although a belief in the possibility of beneficial change may be a sufficient starting point.
Osteopathy	Osteopathy is an established system of diagnosis and treatment that emphasises the structural and functional integrity of the body. The osteopath believes that if the body is functioning to the best of its ability, then its own in-built healing mechanism can function effectively. This will promote long-term health and well-being, while alleviating any existing symptoms. The prime focus of most osteopaths is the musculoskeletal system muscles, bones and joints, which are vital to the healthy functioning of the body as a whole, though some osteopaths also work on internal organs ('visceral osteopathy'). Osteopathy is primarily a manual treatment (though some osteopaths supplement this with the use of ultrasound, etc.). Important is the fine determination of the quality of tissues, or the movement of joint by feel (palpation).

'I trained as a nurse at St George's Hospital in London where I worked for two years after graduating. My interest in acupuncture originates from travelling for two years in China. I completed a three-year course in Traditional Chinese Medicine in 1992 to gain a Licentiate in Acupuncture from the British College of Acupuncture. Then I married and moved to Bristol in 1995 and have been practising acupuncture from home whilst working as a midwife, bringing both skills together where possible.'

Ana

Other therapies used within the NHS include:

Guided imagery	This technique uses the power of mind and imagination to help the patient change their perspective, e.g. to manage stress or to develop a more positive attitude to their illness and healing processes.
Reflexology	Reflexology is a complementary therapy that works on the feet or hands, enabling the body to heal itself. Following illness, stress, injury or disease, the body is in a state of 'imbalance', and vital energy pathways are blocked, preventing it from functioning effectively. Reflexology can be used to restore and maintain the body's natural equilibrium and encourage healing. A reflexologist uses hands only to apply pressure to the feet. For each person the application and the effect of the therapy are unique. Sensitive, trained hands can detect tiny deposits and imbalances in the feet, and by working on these points the reflexologist can release blockages and restore the free flow of energy to the whole body. Tensions are eased, and circulation and elimination is improved. This gentle therapy encourages the body to heal itself, often counteracting a lifetime of misuse.
Relaxation training	Relaxation training focuses on practical techniques such as Autogenic Training and breathing techniques to help someone manage stress.

TRAINING FOR MEDICAL PRACTITIONERS

'We recommend that the UKCC work with the Royal College of Nursing to make CAM (complementary and alternative medicine) familiarisation a part of the undergraduate nursing curriculum and a standard competency expected of

qualified nurses, so that they are aware of the choices that their patients may make. We would also expect nurses specialising in areas where CAM is especially relevant (such as palliative care) to be made aware of any CAM issues particularly pertinent to that speciality during their postgraduate training.

'This is something that the Royal College of Nursing indicated was already beginning, a move we find encouraging. We have no expectation that training in the use of any CAM therapy should be a standard part of a nurse's undergraduate training and would therefore expect that nurses who wish to practise CAM therapies would take up such training post-registration. The Royal College of Nursing and the UKCC, as they do not provide CAM training themselves, should compile a list of courses in CAM that they approve, in order that nurses who wish to practise in this field can obtain guidance on appropriate training.'

UK Government and RCN Guidelines

COMPLEMENTARY THERAPIES IN NURSING AND MIDWIFERY

Complementary Therapies in Nursing and Midwifery is a journal published four times a year and integrates complementary therapies into conventional nursing practices. The journal's coverage includes:

- aromatherapy
- massage
- acupuncture
- reflexology
- herbal medicine.

Complementary Therapies in Nursing and Midwifery's regular features include papers on individual therapies, original research, educational issues, best practice reports and book reviews. Published by: www.harcourt-international.com/journals/ctnm.

Complementary therapies are a major influence on healthcare. Many people use them as an alternative to conventional medicine, but there is an increasing trend towards integrated healthcare where both conventional and complementary therapies are used to benefit the patient. Not only can they work effectively together, but they also provide the patient with a greater sense of control over their own healthcare.

So, not only can you train for a conventional career in health, but you can also bolt on the exciting, practical and fascinating option of a complementary health discipline to truly make you a holistic healthcare practitioner.

If you're a qualified nurse or midwife, you may know all this already. Have you been away from the profession to bring up a family or for a career break? Do you want to return to the healthcare profession fold but are unsure of the next move? Then you need to read the next chapter.

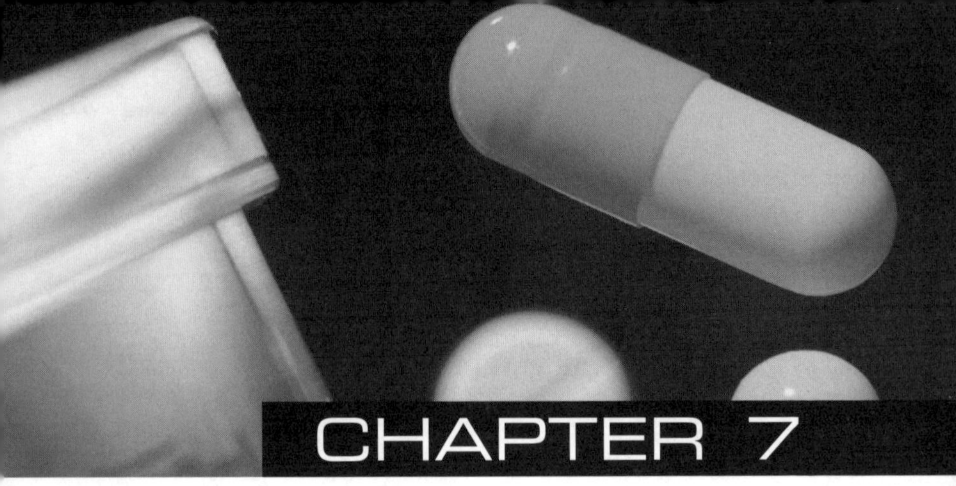

CHAPTER 7

Returning to nursing, midwifery and health visiting

You may have noticed the recent campaign running nationally and backed by local initiatives, to encourage people into or to return to the NHS. The Government is committed to improving the delivery and quality of care to all client/patient groups, and is therefore looking to recruit approximately 15,000 nurses to the NHS within the next three years. You may have been out of the NHS for a period of time, for any of a variety of reasons, including unsocial working hours, bringing up a family, low pay, or inadequate resources. Over the next three years nearly £18 billion is to be invested in the NHS. At the same time, many changes are being introduced to meet the needs of a changing population, including some of the following.

PRIMARY HEALTHCARE GROUPS

Nurses and other professional carers have the opportunity of taking lead roles in developing these groups, which assess, plan and deliver the care required to meet local needs.

NURSES-LED CLINICS

These give another dimension to the nurse's role whilst utilising the skills nurses, midwives and health visitors have in delivering specific care. You could find yourself working in one of the new Health Action Zones.

COMMUNITY SETTINGS

Patients/clients are receiving care at home more often today than ever before. For example, the 'Hospital at Home' scheme allows people to be cared for in their own surroundings whilst receiving vital nursing care.

BENEFITS OF WORKING IN THE NEW NHS

- Employers are being encouraged to introduce family-friendly working with flexible hours. Changes in maternity leave, up to three months' parental leave and leave for domestic crisis are all part of recent legislation.
- The career structure is being altered and will in future allow for better career progression, fairer rewards for team working, developing new skills and taking on extended roles. It will be easier for people to progress whilst staying in practice. The structure will include the new consultant post for nurses, midwives and health visitors.
- Action is being developed to reduce discrimination within the NHS on grounds of gender, race, religion and disability.
- The NHS still offers one of the best occupational pension schemes in the country.
- Up to six weeks' annual leave is available.
- Employment is available in all areas of the country.
- Approved return-to-practice courses are free to potential returners to the NHS.

RETURNING TO PRACTICE ONLINE

Stirling University is planning to set up an online Return to Practice course that will allow nurses to cover all the theoretical aspects of the training they need without ever leaving their homes.

The online course should be especially useful to nurses living in remote rural areas. Once they have finished it, they will then carry out the practical part of their training in work placements in their home area. The website will be run from the university's Highland campus at Inverness.

Isobel Chisholm, a nursing lecturer at Inverness, said she expected the course to be in high demand. 'Our equivalent residential course has always been over-subscribed,' she said.

The NMC requires all nurses, midwives and health visitors whose registration has lapsed for more than five years to undertake a return to practice course before they can be re-admitted to the register.

HOW DO I GET BACK INTO THE NHS?

If you have been working recently and are currently registered to practise as a nurse, midwife or health visitor contact your local NHS Trust HR or personnel department about possible vacancies and opportunities. If you have practised for a while, and your registration has lapsed, you will need to undertake a Return to Practice course. These courses are run nationwide throughout the year. They consist of periods of theory and practice and can last for between 113 and 150 hours depending upon your own need for updating. More courses are becoming available on a part-time basis, and some may be tailor-made to meet your needs. Courses are currently free to the returner.

I AM A SEN NURSE WISHING TO RETURN AND CONVERT TO A FIRST-LEVEL REGISTRATION

You can undertake a conversion course to first-level registration. Courses are usually a minimum of 12 months. This will include theoretical work and a period of supervised practice. It may also give you the opportunity to change specialities in nursing. Courses can often be tailor-made to meet your needs. If you have been out of professional practice for more than a year you may be entitled to a bursary or financial help through the New Deal arrangements.

REGISTRATION

Before you can practise you must have current registration with the NMC. If you have any queries about your registration status, contact the NMC registration department on 020 7333 9333, fax: 020 7333 6561 or email: update@nmc-uk.org

For further information on the above please contact NHS Careers: 0845 60 60 655.

RETURN TO MIDWIFERY PRACTICE

Midwives who have practised for less than 100 days (750 hours) in the five years prior to the renewal of their registration must undertake a return to practice programme. If you are a midwife wanting to return to practice you should:

- speak with a Supervisor of Midwives to identify the length of time you need in practice prior to returning to practice. You can contact a Supervisor through your local maternity unit
- speak with the Head of Midwifery leading the maternity services in the locality in which you hope to practise
- speak with a midwife teacher leading a return to practice programme to outline your study needs – if necessary, consider a return to study programme that would help with the theoretical aspects of the programme. Most higher education institutions that offer midwifery training also provide the theoretical input for return to practice programmes.

WHAT IS THE ROYAL COLLEGE OF MIDWIVES DOING ABOUT RETURN TO PRACTICE FOR MIDWIVES?

The RCM in collaboration with the RCN, undertook a qualitative study, completed in June 2000, which examined the experience of midwives returning to practice. This was funded by the Department of Health, England. One of the key findings of the report was that there needed to be a more co-ordinated approach to the provision of the theory and practice experience for midwives returning to practice.

The RCM approached the Department of Health for funding to support the development of a more flexible process to enable midwives to return to practice. Funding was provided to the RCM for the development of open learning material, in collaboration with the Open University. This programme is the outcome of the development. It has been validated for use in England at both diploma and degree level by Sheffield Hallam University.

The programme comes in a user-friendly distance learning pack. It consists of four main workbooks: *Working in the Modern NHS, Working with Women and Families, Responding to Particular Health and Social Care Needs* and *The Practice Environment*.

There is also a mentor's guide for supporting return to practice midwives in the clinical environment, a study guide and a book of learning resources. For further information please contact Carol Bates, the RCM education development co-ordinator, email: carol.bates@rcm.org.uk.

What do you do next? Turn the page of course.

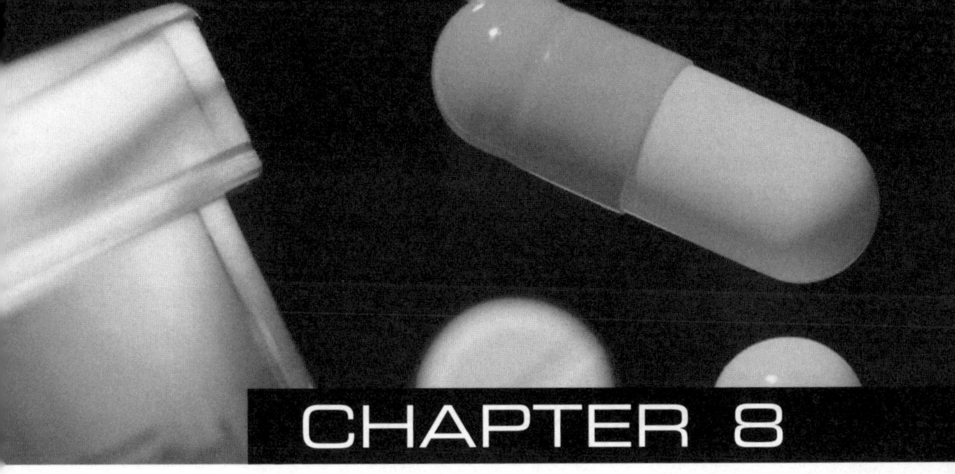

What next?

So where do you go now? What's your next move? Have a look down these options and see what you fancy.

FOR CAREERS INFORMATION

- Independent Midwives Association (IMA). Andrea Dombrowe, 1 The Great Quarry, Guildford, Surrey GU1 3XN. Tel: 01483 821104
- The Nursing and Midwifery Council (NMC), 23 Portland Place, London W1B 1PZ. Tel: 020 7637 7181. Website: www.nmc-uk.org
- NHS Careers: PO Box 376, Bristol BS99 3EY. Tel: 0845 606 0655. Website: www.nhscareers.nhs.uk. NHS Careers provides advice and information on all careers in the NHS in the UK. It also has a database of all universities that provide midwifery courses
- Royal College of Nursing, 20 Cavendish Road, London W1M 0AB. Tel: 020 7409 3333. Website: www.rcn.org.uk
- Royal College of Midwives, 15 Mansfield Street, London W1G 9NH. Tel: 020 7312 3535. Website: www.rcm.org.uk

- Community Practitioners and Health Visitors Association, 40 Bermondsey Street, London SE1 3UD. Tel: 020 7939 7000. Website: www.amicus-cphva.org

- Read *Careers in Nursing and Related Professions* by Linda Nazarko, published by Kogan page.

IF YOU'RE READY TO APPLY FOR TRAINING

- Read *The Directory of Nursing and Midwifery Courses,* published by Trotman

- Applying for diploma programmes:

  Nursing & Midwifery Admissions Service (NMAS), Rosehill, New Barn Lane, Cheltenham, Gloucestershire GL52 3LZ. Tel: 0870 112 2200 (applications). Tel: 0870 112 2206 (general enquiries). Website: www.nmas.ac.uk

- Applying for degree programmes:

  Universities & Colleges Admissions Service (UCAS), Rosehill, New Barn Lane, Cheltenham, Gloucestershire GL52 3LZ. Tel: 0870 112 2200 (applications). Tel: 0870 112 2211 (general enquiries). Website: www.ucas.ac.uk

- For visa queries for applicants from non-EEA countries contact:

  Immigration & Nationality Directorate, The Home Office, Lunar House, 40 Wellesley Road, Croydon CR9 2BY. Tel: 0870 606 7766.

- For queries relating to bursaries and financial support contact:

  The NHS Student Grants Unit, 22 Plymouth Road, Blackpool FY3 7JS. Tel: 01253 655655. Email: nhs-sgu@ukonline.co.uk.

Ready for your next move? Take it now and good luck with your new career in nursing or midwifery.